National Health Statistics Reports

Number 34 ■ May 19, 2011

An Overview of Home Health Aides: United States, 2007

by Anita Bercovitz, M.P.H., Ph.D.; Abigail Moss; Manisha Sengupta, Ph.D.; Eunice Y. Park-Lee; Ph.D.; Adrienne Jones; and Lauren D. Harris-Kojetin, Ph.D., Division of Health Care Statistics, National Center for Health Statistics; and Marie R. Squillace, Ph.D., Office of the Assistant Secretary for Planning and Evaluation, U.S. Department of Health and Human Services

Abstract

Objectives—This report presents national estimates of home health aides providing assistance in activities of daily living (ADLs) and employed by agencies providing home health and hospice care in 2007. Data are presented on demographics, training, work environment, pay and benefits, use of public benefits, and injuries.

Methods—Estimates are based on data collected in the 2007 National Home Health Aide Survey. Estimates are derived from data collected during telephone interviews with home health aides providing assistance with ADLs and employed by agencies providing home health and hospice care.

Results—In the United States in 2007, 160,700 home health and hospice aides provided ADL assistance and were employed by agencies providing home health and hospice care. Most home health aides were female; approximately one-half were white and one-third black. Approximately one-half of aides were at least 35 years old. Two-thirds had an annual family income of less than $40,000. More than 80% received initial training to become a home health aide and more than 90% received continuing education classes in the previous 2 years. Almost three-quarters of aides would definitely become a home health aide again, and slightly more than one-half of aides would definitely take their current job again. The average hourly pay was $10.88 per hour. Almost three-quarters of aides reported that they were offered health insurance by their employers, but almost 19% of aides had no health insurance coverage from any source. More than 1 in 10 aides had had at least one work-related injury in the previous 12 months.

Conclusions—The picture that emerges from this analysis is of a financially vulnerable workforce, but one in which the majority of aides are satisfied with their jobs. The findings may be useful in informing initiatives to train, recruit, and retain these direct care workers.

Keywords: direct care worker • National Home Health Aide Survey • hospice aide • long-term care

Introduction

By 2050, the estimated number of persons who will need some type of long-term care is projected to almost double—from 15 million in 2000 to 27 million, assuming current patterns of care continue (1). Of those, the majority will receive long-term care in the community rather than in institutions. Currently, the majority of home- and community-based long-term care is provided by unpaid caregivers, such as family members, neighbors, or friends. Although unpaid care remains the primary source of community-based long-term care, the demand for paid (formal) caregivers is expected to increase (1). The bulk of formal long-term care is provided by direct care workers, such as nursing assistants, home health aides, and personal aides, who provide basic care and essential help with daily activities, enabling people with functional and activity limitations to live independently in their homes.

In 2006, about 3 million people were employed in the direct care industry, including nursing, psychiatric, and home health aides. Direct care jobs are projected to be among the fastest-growing occupations in the near future, with the greatest increases among home

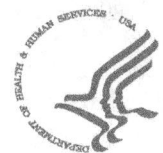

U.S. DEPARTMENT OF HEALTH AND HUMAN SERVICES
Centers for Disease Control and Prevention
National Center for Health Statistics

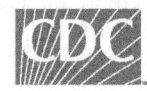

health aides. Projected employment of home health aides is expected to increase 50% between 2008 and 2018—from 921,000 to 1,382,000 (2).

Given the projected demand for direct care workers, recruitment of additional workers and retention of currently employed workers is crucial. Retention of direct care workers is a major challenge. A low pay structure, lack of or limited fringe benefits, a heavy workload, poor working conditions, lack of appropriate training, little opportunity for professional advancement, and a lack of respect from management are some of the reasons cited for high turnover and vacancy rates (3,4). National data on direct care workers are limited, as most of the few existing studies are restricted to smaller geographic areas. The Bureau of Labor Statistics (BLS) provides estimates of employment in the home health aide industry to monitor labor force participation (5). However, no nationally representative data are collected from home health aides that could provide their perspectives on the work environment, job satisfaction, and retention. Given the high turnover and vacancy rates (6), these data could help policymakers understand the needs of and challenges faced by home health aides, and identify strategies that can enhance the home health aide experience.

Recognizing the need to fill the gap in data about factors related to recruitment and retention of home health aides, the Department of Health and Human Services' Office of the Assistant Secretary for Planning and Evaluation (ASPE) sponsored the National Home Health Aide Survey (NHHAS). NHHAS provides the first nationally representative data source on home health aides employed by agencies providing home health or hospice care. This report presents estimates on home health aides' demographics and employing agency characteristics; aides' reasons for becoming aides and attitudes toward their jobs; training; work environment; pay, employer-offered benefits, and use of public benefits; and work-related injuries. These estimates help paint a picture of home health

aides—a crucial group of direct care workers providing long-term care.

Methods

Data source

Data are from NHHAS, the first nationally representative sample survey of home health aides. NHHAS, a two-stage probability sample survey, was a supplement to the 2007 National Home and Hospice Care Survey (NHHCS) conducted by the Centers for Disease Control and Prevention's National Center for Health Statistics in partnership with ASPE. Agencies providing home health or hospice care were sampled for NHHCS, then aides were sampled from participating sampled NHHCS agencies. Aides who were directly employed by the sampled agency and provided assistance in activities of daily living (ADLs)—including eating, toileting, bathing, dressing, or transferring—were eligible to participate in NHHAS. Aides were interviewed using computer-assisted telephone interviewing or CATI technology. Data collection was conducted by Westat. NHHAS data collection is authorized under Section 306 of the Public Health Service Act (Title 42 U.S. Code, 242K).

For further information on the sampling, survey design, and other survey methodology, see "Technical Notes" in this report, documentation available from http://www.cdc.gov/nchs/nhhas.htm, or *Vital and Health Statistics* Series 1, Number 49 (7).

Data analysis

All analyses were performed in SAS-callable SUDAAN (8) to account for sampling weights and the complex sampling design. In some tables, categories were collapsed to permit reporting of reliable estimates.

Chi-square tests and *t* tests were used to test for significance at the $p < 0.05$ level. *T* tests were not adjusted for multiple comparisons. The difference between any two estimates is mentioned in the text only if it is statistically significant and represents an absolute

difference of at least 10 percentage points. This approach is intended to highlight meaningful differences. Terms such as "similar" or "no significant differences" are used to denote that the estimates being compared are not significantly different statistically. Comparisons not mentioned may or may not be statistically significant.

Nonresponse was handled differently for different variables. Missing values for age, sex, and race were imputed using the hot-deck method. Nonresponse for these variables was 1.8% for age, 1.36% for sex, and 1.64% for race. Nonresponses (e.g., "don't know" and "refused") were excluded when calculating estimates for other continuous variables (e.g., hourly wage and agency size based on number of current patients). The percentage of cases with nonresponses for continuous variables ranged from 4.8% for agency size to 6.7% for hourly wage. For other categorical variables, nonresponses were recoded as unknown and included in the analyses. The percentage of nonresponse for categorical variables ranged from 1.36% for sex to 14.5% for the aide's response to whether the agency offered paid or subsidized child care. When 5% or more of the responses were unknown, an "unknown" category was included in the tables. When an unknown category has less than 5% nonresponse, the unknown category is not reported in the tables. Unknowns are included in the denominators for percent distribution estimates regardless of the percentages unknown and whether they are or are not reported in the table. Except where noted, figures depicting percentages also include the unknown category in the denominator, even when the unknown category itself is not depicted in the figure. For this reason, category-specific sample sizes may sum to less than table or figure totals, and percent distributions may sum to less than 100%. Because nonresponses were included in the denominator when calculating percentages, the percentages reported are underestimates.

In this report, the term "aides" is used to refer to home health and hospice aides. Agencies that provided both home health and hospice care are referred to as mixed agencies.

Results

Employer characteristics

- In the United States in 2007, 160,700 home health and hospice aides provided ADL assistance and were employed by agencies providing home health and hospice care (Table 1).
- Almost three-fourths of these aides (74.2%) worked for agencies that provided home health care only.
- More than three-fifths of aides (63.3%) worked for proprietary agencies.
- Almost one-half of aides (47.0%) worked for agencies located in the South.
- Over four-fifths of aides (84.0%) were employed by agencies located in metropolitan areas.
- More than two-thirds of aides (70.0%) worked for independent agencies, that is, agencies that were not part of a chain of agencies.

Aide characteristics

- Little more than one-half of the aides were white (53.3%) and aged 35 years and over (56.5%). An overwhelming majority of the aides were non-Hispanic (90.2%) and female (95.0%).
- More than three-quarters of aides (77.3%) had at least a high school diploma.
- Nearly one-half of all aides (50.3%) were married or living with a partner.
- Almost one-half of all aides (46.9%) had a family income of $30,000 or less.
- Most aides were U.S. citizens (94.2%). Of these, most were citizens by birth (89.6%).

Reasons for becoming aides and whether would become an aide again

- More than three-fourths of aides stated that they became aides because these jobs were available close to where they lived (80.3%), they eventually wanted to become a nurse (80.0%), they had provided care to

friends or relatives (76.7%), or these jobs were steady and secure (76.2%) (Table 2).
- A higher percentage of female aides (81.1%) than male aides (59.5%) became aides because they wanted to eventually become a nurse. On the other hand, more male aides (90.0%) than female aides (73.3%) reported becoming aides because family members or friends were also home health aides.
- Aides aged 25–34 were more likely than those under age 25 to become aides because they provided care to a friend or relative (81.0% compared with 60.9%), and liked helping people (68.5% compared with 47.3%).
- Nearly three-fourths of current aides (72.2%) would definitely become an aide again (Table 3).
- Compared with those aged 45–54 (76.3%) or those aged 55 and over (74.3%), aides under age 25 (49.9%) were less likely to report that they would definitely become an aide again.
- Aides with no high school diploma or General Educational Development (GED) high school equivalency diploma (86.7%) were more likely than those who had some college or trade school (66.6%) to indicate that they would definitely become an aide again.

Training

Initial training

- More than four-fifths of aides (83.9%) had received initial training (Table 4).
- More aides aged 35–44 had taken initial training (89.6%) than aides aged 25–34 (74.4%).
- A greater percentage of aides of other races had taken initial training (95.1%) than white aides (79.1%).
- Aides with less than a high school diploma or GED were more likely to have taken initial training (96.1%) than aides who had a GED (82.4%), a high school diploma (81.4%), or some college (83.9%).

- Among aides who had taken initial training, over four-fifths (82.2%) thought the training prepared them well for their jobs (Table 5).
- Aides whose initial training was either mostly hands-on (81.6%) or evenly split between hands-on and classroom training (87.2%) felt more well-prepared for their jobs than aides whose initial training was mostly classroom study (60.7%).

Continuing education

- Most aides had taken continuing education (91.0%), including in-service training, in the past 2 years (Table 4).
- Aides aged 25–54 were more likely to have taken continuing education in the past 2 years (over 90%) than aides under age 25 (76.6%).
- Among aides who had taken continuing education in the past 2 years, including in-service training, almost four-fifths found the training very useful (79.1%), and about one-fifth found it somewhat or not at all useful (20.9%) (Table 6).
- A higher percentage of aides working in the South (84.9%) found their continuing education very useful compared with aides working in the Midwest (69.9%).
- Aides who said they would definitely become an aide again were more likely than aides who said they would probably become an aide again to rate their continuing education as very useful (86.2% compared with 63.7%).
- Aides who rated their continuing education very useful were more than twice as likely to be extremely satisfied with their jobs as aides who rated their continuing education somewhat or not at all useful (52.3% compared with 22.7%) (Figure 1).
- Conversely, aides who found their continuing education somewhat or not at all useful were more than three times as likely to be dissatisfied with their jobs as aides who rated their continuing education very useful (25.9% compared with 7.5%).

Work environment

- Over two-thirds of aides (69.6%) reported the number of hours they

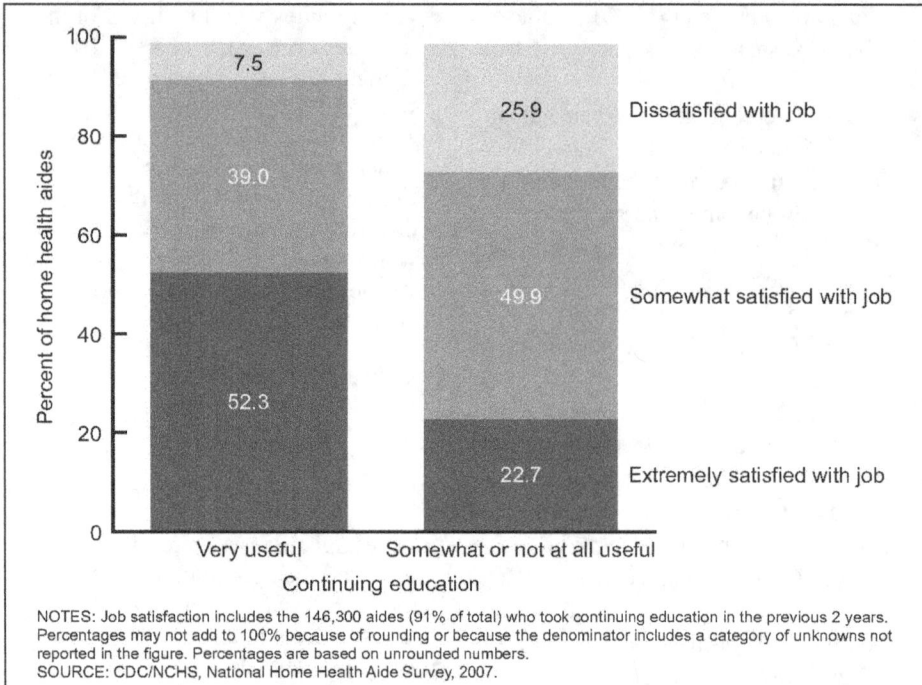

Figure 1. Usefulness of continuing education, by job satisfaction: United States, 2007

NOTES: Job satisfaction includes the 146,300 aides (91% of total) who took continuing education in the previous 2 years. Percentages may not add to 100% because of rounding or because the denominator includes a category of unknowns not reported in the figure. Percentages are based on unrounded numbers.
SOURCE: CDC/NCHS, National Home Health Aide Survey, 2007.

worked was about right; however, about one-quarter of aides (26.2%) would prefer to work more hours (Table 7).

- More than 90% of aides reported having enough or more than enough time to assist patients with ADLs (Table 8).
- One-half of all aides (50.0%) had worked as a home health aide for 11 years or more, about four-tenths (41.3%) had worked as an aide between 2 and 10 years, and less than one-tenth (8.6%) had worked as an aide fewer than 2 years (Figure 2).
- Slightly over one-third of aides working in micropolitan statistical areas (35.6%) had worked as an aide for 11 years or more, less than aides working in metropolitan statistical areas (51.9%) and aides working in other locations (48.6%) (Table 9).
- The opportunity for career advancement was a reason for continuing in their current job for 89.4% of aides under age 25, cited more than among aides aged 25–34 (71.7%) and aides aged 55 and over (76.0%) (Table 10).
- The opportunity to work overtime was a reason for continuing in their

current job for 47.3% of aides under age 25, cited less frequently than aides aged 25–34 (75.1%), 45–54 (72.4%), and 55 and over (76.5%). The opportunity to work overtime was also cited more frequently as a reason for continuing in their current job among male aides (84.4%) than female aides (70.3%).

- Almost one-half of aides (46.7%) were extremely satisfied with their job, 40.4% were somewhat satisfied, and 11.7% were somewhat or extremely dissatisfied (Table 11).
- Among aides who were extremely satisfied with their job, 77.0% were extremely satisfied with the opportunity to do challenging work, 73.0% were extremely satisfied with their opportunities to learn new skills, 47.0% were extremely satisfied with their benefits, and 31.6% were extremely satisfied with their salary.
- About three-fourths of aides (75.7%) felt their supervisor respected them a great deal as part of the health care team, and 89.6% felt that patients respected them a great deal as part of the health care team.
- Fifty-four percent of aides would definitely take their current job again,

while 14.0% would probably or definitely not take their current job again.

- Virtually all aides felt their work was very important (96.5%). However, fewer aides thought that their supervisors (76.5%), their organizations (66.3%), and society (56.1%) valued their work very much. Aides' perceptions of the three groups' value of their work were all significantly different from each other (Figure 3).

Pay and employer-offered benefits

- During 2007–2008, home health and hospice aides earned, on average, $10.88 per hour (Table 12). The federal minimum wage rate specified in the Fair Labor Standards Act that went into effect July 24, 2007, was $5.85 (available from http:// www.laborlawcenter.com/t-federal-minimum-wage.aspx).
- Aides working in areas outside of metropolitan and micropolitan statistical areas had the lowest average hourly wage ($8.12 per hour), compared with $10.91 per hour in metropolitan and $12.16 per hour in micropolitan statistical areas.
- More than one-half of all aides (56.7%) received a pay raise during the past year.
- Aides working for home health care only agencies were less likely to receive a pay raise within the past year (51.6%) than aides working for hospice care only (69.6%) and mixed agencies (73.3%).
- Aides working for home health care only agencies were less likely to be offered health insurance benefits (66.0%) than were aides working for hospice care only (94.3%) and mixed agencies (89.2%) (Table 13 and Figure 4).
- Over one-half of aides worked for agencies that offered extra pay for working holidays (62.0%) or other paid time off (59.1%); dental, vision, or drug benefits (56.0%); disability or life insurance (53.2%); or paid holidays (51.2%) or paid sick leave (50.5%).

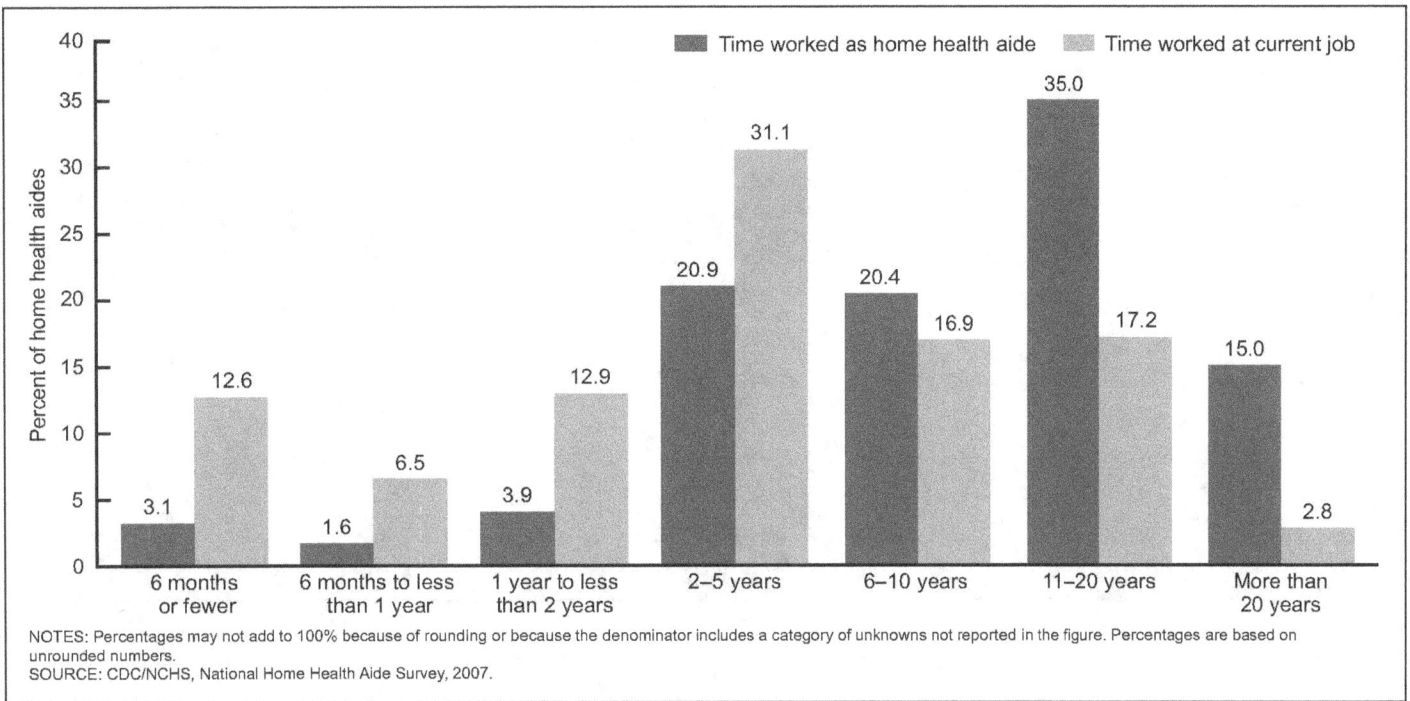

Figure 2. Length of time worked as home health aide and at current job: United States, 2007

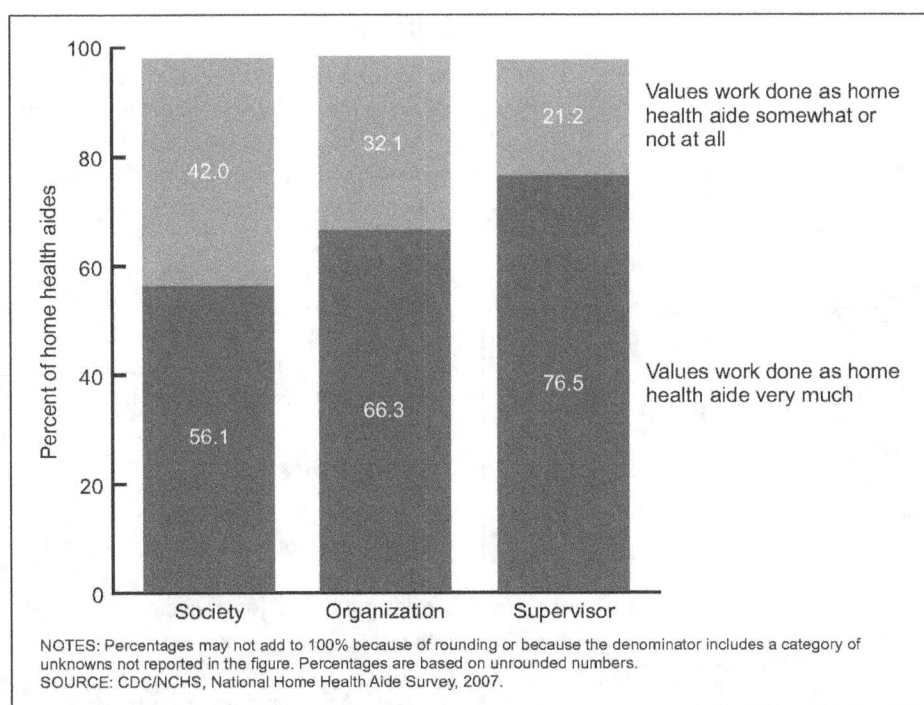

Figure 3. Home health aides' perception of how others value their work: United States, 2007

- About two-thirds of aides working in large home health care only agencies received dental, vision, or drug benefits (66.3%), compared with about one-third of aides in medium (32.7%) and about one-quarter of aides in smaller agencies (23.6%) of this type.
- While about three-fourths of all aides were offered health insurance by their

employers (72.7%), only about one-third of all aides enrolled in their employers' plans (37.5%) (Table 14).

- Among all aides, about one-third had health insurance coverage that was exclusively provided by their employer (31.9%), and about one-tenth had more than one source of health insurance (11.1%), including employer and nonemployer sources. Almost one-fifth of all aides had no health insurance coverage (18.8%) through their employer, spouse or another individual, or a government plan, such as Medicaid or Medicare (Figure 5).

Use of public benefits

- Slightly over one-half of all aides (51.8%) had received benefits prior to or were receiving benefits at the time of the NHHAS from at least one of the following programs: Temporary Assistance for Needy Families (TANF); Special Supplemental Nutrition Program for Women, Infants, and Children (WIC); or food stamps (Table 15).
- Almost one-tenth of aides were receiving benefits from at least one of

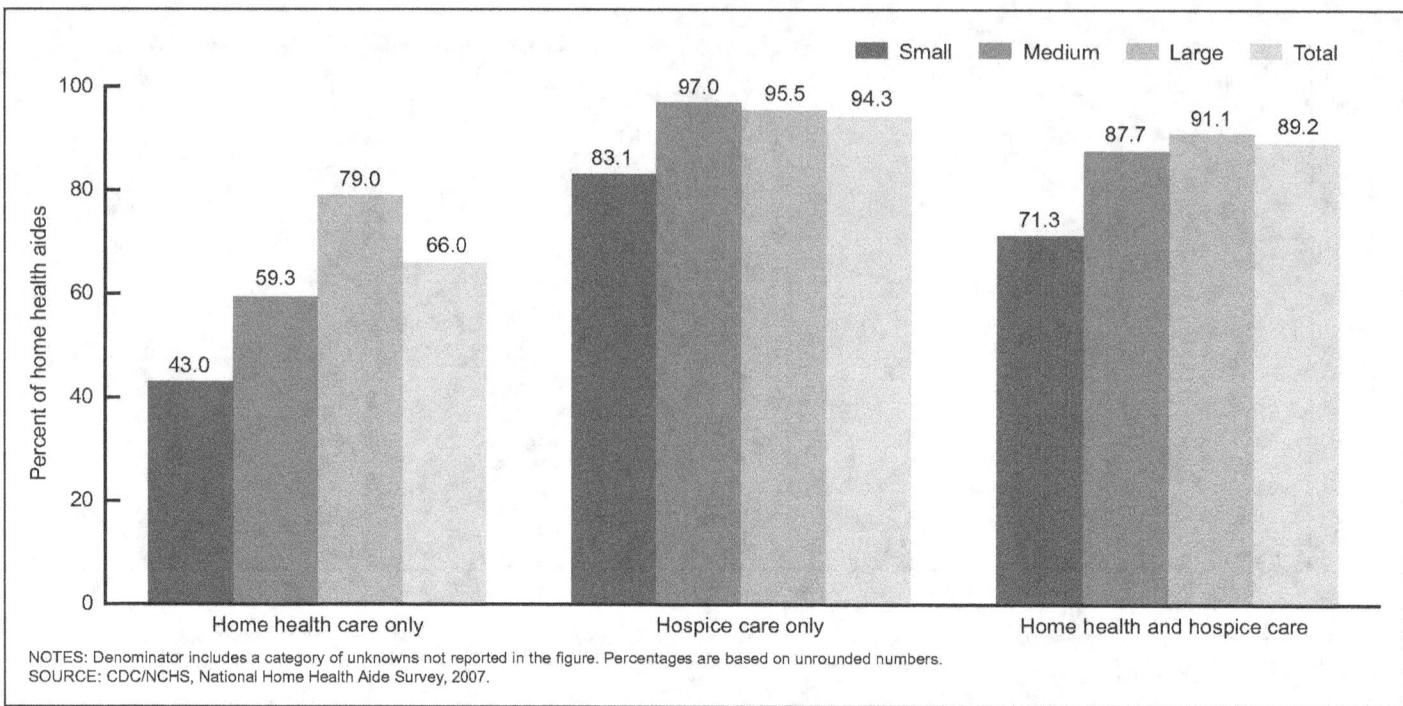

Figure 4. Home health aides employed by agencies offering health insurance, by agency type and size: United States, 2007

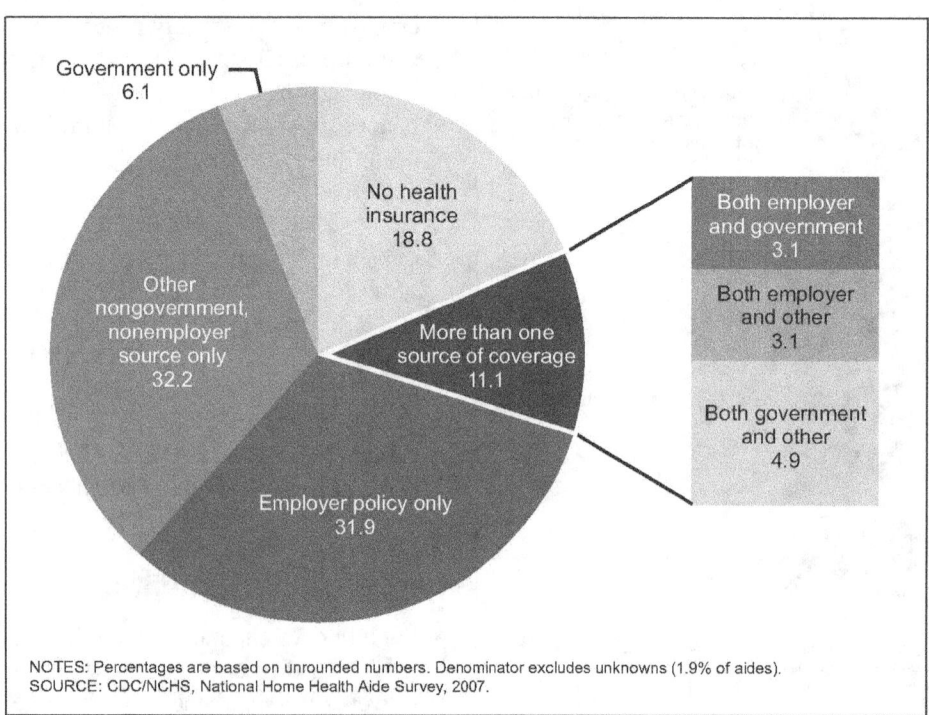

NOTES: Percentages are based on unrounded numbers. Denominator excludes unknowns (1.9% of aides).
SOURCE: CDC/NCHS, National Home Health Aide Survey, 2007.

Figure 5. Source of health insurance for home health aides: United States, 2007

Injuries

- At least one work-related injury in the previous 12 months was reported by 11.5% of aides (Table 16).
- Among aides with injuries, 83.4% had only one injury.
- Back injuries (44.3%) and other strains or pulled muscles (43.2%) were the two most common types of injuries reported among the aides with one or more work-related injuries in the past 12 months.

Discussion

These data are based on self-reports through telephone interviews with 3,377 aides providing assistance in ADLs, working directly for agencies providing home health or hospice care and employed by the agency at the time of the NHHAS. The data from the first nationally representative sample of home health aides are especially useful because they are based on direct interviews with the aides. Aides are part of a workforce where demand is expected to increase, and supply is expected to be insufficient to meet demand (2). NHHAS data can be useful as a basis for developing approaches for

these programs (9.9%) at the time of NHHAS.
- Among all aides, 5.4% were receiving housing assistance (rental subsidy, lower rent because of government contributions, or living in public housing) at the time of the interview.

improving work experiences and increasing recruitment and retention. The results presented in this report are similar to studies of other direct care workers (4,9,10) but also provide a more complete picture of aides' work experiences and attitudes toward their jobs.

Home health aides' demographics are not representative of the U.S. population overall. The majority of aides are female. While the majority of aides are white, 34.9% of aides are black—more than twice the percentage in the 2007 U.S. population (13.5% of the U.S. population identified as black alone or in combination with other races, with 12.8% identified as black alone) (11). The percentage of aides with at least a high school diploma or GED was 92.8%, compared with 84% in the U.S. population aged 25 and over in 2007. However, the percentage of aides with a college or advanced degree was 5.9% compared with 27.5% for the U.S. population aged 25 and over (12).

Almost one-half of all aides had a total family income of $30,000 or less, compared with a 2007 national median family income of $50,233 (13). Aides reported a mean of $10.88 per hour (median $10.51) compared with national estimates of $10.03 (median $9.62) reported by BLS for 2007 for home health aides. The national mean and median hourly wage estimates for all occupations were $19.56 (mean) and $15.10 (median), and for health care support occupations were $12.31 (mean) and $11.45 (median) in 2007 (14). Seventeen percent of aides were extremely satisfied with their salaries, and 43.5% were somewhat satisfied with their salaries, while 37.8% were somewhat or extremely dissatisfied.

Most aides reported working for agencies that offered a variety of benefits, including health insurance and paid time off. The most common benefit aides reported was health insurance. Although 72.7% of aides worked for agencies that offered health insurance, only 37.5% of aides enrolled in the employer plan. Most aides whose agency did not offer health insurance or did not enroll in the agency plan were covered by a spouse's plan, purchased

coverage on their own, or were covered by a government plan. Almost one-fifth of aides were not covered by any health insurance (18.5%) compared with 15% of the population nationwide in 2007 (13). Among those aides offered health insurance by their employer, 11.9% were not covered by any other plan. The Affordable Care Act (P.L. 111–148) expands insurance coverage and makes coverage more affordable. Thus, home health aides who are currently uninsured may have the opportunity to obtain health insurance. NHHAS data provide a baseline of the prevalence of health insurance coverage among home health aides prior to implementation of the new law.

More than one-half of aides worked for agencies that they reported offered some type of paid time off, including paid vacation or personal days (59.1%), paid holidays (51.2%), or sick leave (50.5%). Other common benefits included extra pay for working holidays (62.0%); dental, vision, or drug benefits (56.0%); and/or disability or life insurance (53.2%). While over one-half of aides reported that they were either extremely (28.5%) or somewhat satisfied (28.9%) with the job benefits, 37.8% were either somewhat or extremely dissatisfied.

More than one-half of aides had received TANF, WIC, or food stamps at some point prior to the NHHAS, and one-tenth of aides were receiving benefits from one or more of those programs at the time of the survey. Forty percent of aides had received WIC at some point prior to the NHHAS, and 4.8% were receiving WIC at the time of the survey, compared with 3.4% of women of childbearing age (15–44 years) in 2007, based on national population estimates and WIC program data (15). Among aides, 41.8% had received food stamps prior to the NHHAS, and 6.7% were receiving food stamps at time of the survey, compared with 7.7% of U.S households in 2007 that received food stamps or benefits from the Supplemental Nutrition Assistance Program (SNAP), as reported by the Department of Commerce (16). Since the percentages presented in this report are calculated with a denominator

including all aides, not just aides eligible for these benefits, these percentages underestimate the percentage of qualified aides receiving benefits.

In 2007, home health aides were experienced and committed to the field of home health care and to their current job. One-half of all aides had worked as an aide for 10 years or more, and 15.0% had worked as an aide for more than 20 years. Seventy-two percent of aides would definitely become an aide again—a measure of commitment to the field of home health care, and 84.5% would probably or definitely take their current job again—a measure of commitment to their current job. Older home health aides were more likely than younger aides to say they would become an aide again. Virtually all aides felt their work was very important (96.5%), but their perception of how others valued their work varied. Slightly over three-quarters of aides felt that their supervisor valued their work very much, and aides felt that 66.3% of the organizations they work for value their work very much.

Recent legislation, including the Affordable Care Act and the American Recovery and Reinvestment Act (P.L. 111–5), included provisions to fund training for direct care workers in long-term care settings. Most aides had both initial training and continuing education. More than 80% of aides received some initial training, and of those, 82.0% felt this training left them well-prepared for the reality of working in home health care. Over 90% of aides received some continuing education in the 2 years prior to the NHHAS, and 79.1% of those aides found the training very useful.

Home health aides' reasons for becoming and staying aides were predominantly practical but varied by age. The most common reasons cited for becoming an aide were related both to interest in health care (wanting to become a nurse) and pragmatic interests (jobs were close to home and job was steady and secure). Life and family experiences were also commonly cited reasons for becoming aides: either the aide provided care to family or friends, or family or friends were also aides. The reasons that aides cited most frequently for continuing to work in their current job included career advancement opportunities, the opportunity to work overtime, working with a care team, and enjoying caring for others. Aides under age 25 were more likely than older aides to say they stayed in their jobs because of opportunities for career advancement but less likely to stay because of the opportunity to work overtime. Almost 90% of aides were either extremely or somewhat satisfied with their current job, but their level of satisfaction varied by aspect. While more than one-half of aides were extremely satisfied with opportunities for doing challenging work (59.1%) and with learning new skills (56.0%), only 28.5% were extremely satisfied with their benefits, and 17.2% were extremely satisfied with their salary. The majority thought the number of hours they worked was about right (69.6%) and that they either had more than enough or enough time to provide ADL assistance to their patients (93.4%).

The picture that emerges from this analysis is of a financially vulnerable workforce, with low family income, a large percentage that currently or previously received public benefits, almost one-fifth without health insurance, and more than 1 in 10 having a least one work-related injury in the past year. At the same time, the majority of aides are satisfied with their job overall, would definitely become an aide again, and feel the work they do is valuable and rewarding. In light of the projected demand for home health aides, these findings from the NHHAS may be useful in informing initiatives to train, recruit, and retain these direct care workers.

References

1. U.S. Department of Health and Human Services, U.S. Department of Labor. The future supply of long-term care workers in relation to the aging baby boom generation: Report to Congress. Washington, DC. 2003. Available from: http://aspe.hhs.gov/daltcp/reports/ltcwork.htm [Accessed 7/12/10].

2. U.S. Department of Labor, Bureau of Labor Statistics. Selected occupational projections data. Available from: http://data.bls.gov/oep/noeted [Accessed 1/31/11].

3. Institute of Medicine of the National Academies. Retooling for an aging America: Building the health care workforce. Washington, DC: The National Academies Press. 2008.

4. Hewitt A, Larson S, Edelstein S, Seavey D, Hoge MA, Morris J. A synthesis of direct service workforce demographics and challenges across intellectual/developmental disabilities, aging, physical disabilities, and behavioral health. National Direct Service Workforce Resource Center. 2008. Available from: http://www.directcare clearinghouse.org/l_art_det.jsp?res_id=292110 [Accessed 7/12/10].

5. U.S. Department of Labor, Bureau of Labor Statistics. Occupational outlook handbook, 2010-11 edition. Available from: http://www.bls.gov/oco/ocos326.htm [Accessed 7/12/10].

6. Stone RI, Wiener JM. Who will care for us? Addressing the long-term care workforce crisis. Urban Institute and American Association of Homes and Services for the Aging. 2001. Available from: http://www.urban.org/publications/310304.html [Accessed 7/12/10].

7. Bercovitz A, Moss AJ, Sengupta M, et al. Design and operation of the National Home Health Aide Survey: 2007–2008. National Center for Health Statistics. Vital Health Stat 1(49). 2010.

8. Research Triangle Institute. SUDAAN (Release 9.1.1). Research Triangle Park, NC. 2005.

9. Yamada Y. Profile of home care aides, nursing home aides, and hospital aides: Historical changes and data recommendations. Gerontologist 42(2):199–206. 2002.

10. Montgomery RJ, Holley L, Deichert J, Kosloski K. A profile of home care workers from the 2000 census: How it changes what we know. Gerontologist 45(5):593–600. 2005.

11. U.S. Census Bureau. Population estimates: National - characteristics: National sex, race, and Hispanic origin. Table 3: Annual estimates of the population by sex, race and Hispanic origin for the United States: April 1, 2000 to July 1, 2007. Available from: http://www.census.gov/popest/national/asrh/NC-EST2007-srh.html [Accessed 7/12/10].

12. Crissey SR. Educational attainment in the United States: 2007. Current population reports, P20–560. Washington, DC: U.S. Census Bureau. 2009. Available from: http://www.census.gov/prod/2009pubs/p20-560.pdf [Accessed 7/12/10].

13. DeNavas-Walt C, Proctor BD, Smith JC. Income, poverty, and health insurance coverage in the United States: 2007. Current population reports, P60–235. Washington, DC: U.S. Census Bureau. 2008. Available from: http://www.census.gov/prod/2007pubs/p60-233.pdf [Accessed 7/12/10].

14. U.S. Department of Labor, Bureau of Labor Statistics. Occupational employment statistics: May 2007 national occupational employment and wage estimates, United States. 2007. Available from: http://www.bls.gov/oes/2007/may/oes_nat.htm [Accessed 7/12/10].

15. U.S. Department of Agriculture. WIC program monthly data: Special supplemental nutrition program for women, infants and children (WIC)—2007. Available from: http://www.fns.usda.gov/pd/37WIC_Monthly.htm [Accessed 7/12/10].

16. Loveless TA. Food stamp/supplemental nutrition assistance program (SNAP) receipt in the past 12 months for households: 2008 American Community Survey. American Community Survey reports, ACSBR/08–8. Washington, DC: U.S. Census Bureau. 2009. Available from: http://www.census.gov/prod/2009pubs/acsbr08-8.pdf [Accessed 7/12/10].

17. Dwyer LL, Harris-Kojetin LD, Branden L, Shimizu IM. Redesign and operation of the National Home and Hospice Care Survey, 2007. National Center for Health Statistics. Vital Health Stat 1(53). 2010.

Table 1. Employer and aide characteristics of currently employed home health aides: United States, 2007

Characteristic	All home health aides			
	Number	Standard error	Percent distribution	Standard error
All home health aides[1]	160,700	11,479	100.0	. . .
Employer characteristic				
Type of care provided:				
Home health care only.	119,200	11,329	74.2	2.6
Hospice care only.	20,000	1,605	12.4	1.3
Home health and hospice care.	21,500	3,372	13.4	2.2
Ownership:				
Proprietary	101,700	10,833	63.3	4.1
Voluntary nonprofit	51,400	6,630	32.0	3.9
Government and other.	†7,600	†2,417	†4.7	†1.5
Geographic region:				
Northeast	23,600	3,979	14.7	2.6
Midwest	49,400	7,529	30.8	4.2
South	75,600	10,541	47.0	4.7
West	12,100	2,340	7.5	1.6
Location:				
Metropolitan statistical area[2]	135,000	11,251	84.0	1.7
Micropolitan statistical area[3]	16,700	2,120	10.4	1.4
Other location	9,000	1,276	5.6	0.9
Chain affiliation:				
Part of a chain.	48,100	6,857	30.0	4.0
Not part of a chain	112,600	11,014	70.0	4.0
Aide characteristic				
Age at time of interview:				
Under 25 years	8,200	1,789	5.1	1.1
25–34 years	25,600	3,286	15.9	1.8
35–44 years	36,100	3,379	22.5	1.8
45–54 years	47,900	4,775	29.8	2.0
55 years and over	42,900	5,062	26.7	2.0
Sex:				
Female	152,700	11,032	95.0	0.9
Male	8,000	1,608	5.0	0.9
Race:				
White	85,700	7,624	53.3	3.3
Black	56,100	6,889	34.9	3.4
Other[4]	18,900	3,514	11.8	1.9
Hispanic or Latino origin:				
Hispanic or Latino.	13,000	2,717	8.1	1.7
Not Hispanic or Latino	144,900	10,980	90.2	1.8
Education:				
No high school diploma or GED certificate[5]	11,500	2,349	7.1	1.4
GED certificate[5]	22,900	3,258	14.2	1.7
High school diploma	60,600	5,563	37.7	2.4
Some college or trade school	54,100	5,004	33.7	1.9
College graduate or postgraduate	9,400	2,361	5.9	1.4
Marital status:				
Married or living with partner	80,800	6,329	50.3	2.6
Widowed, divorced, or separated	51,400	5,314	32.0	2.3
Never married	26,300	3,888	16.4	2.0
Citizenship:				
U.S. citizen.	151,300	10,985	94.1	1.3
By birth	135,500	10,586	84.3	2.2
By naturalization	15,800	3,377	9.8	2.2
Not U.S. citizen	7,200	1,785	4.5	1.1

See footnotes at end of table.

Table 1. Employer and aide characteristics of currently employed home health aides: United States, 2007—Con.

Characteristic	All home health aides			
	Number	Standard error	Percent distribution	Standard error
Family income:				
Less than $20,000	34,500	4,441	21.5	2.2
$20,000–$29,999	40,800	4,428	25.4	2.1
$30,000–$39,999	32,900	3,625	20.5	1.7
$40,000–$49,999	17,300	2,743	10.8	1.5
$50,000 or more	26,700	3,202	16.6	1.8
Unknown	8,400	2,000	5.2†	1.1

. . . Category not applicable.

† Estimate does not meet standards of reliability or precision because the sample size is between 30 and 59, or the sample size is greater than 59 but has a relative standard error of 30% or more.

[1]Includes home health aides currently employed by agencies that provide home health care services, hospice care services, or both types of services, and currently serve or recently served home health or hospice care patients. Agencies that provided only homemaker services or housekeeping services, assistance with instrumental activities of daily living, or durable medical equipment and supplies were excluded from the survey.

[2]A county or group of contiguous counties that contains at least one urbanized area of 50,000 or more population and may contain other counties that are economically and socially integrated with the central county as measured by commuting.

[3]A nonmetropolitan county or group of contiguous nonmetropolitan counties that contains an urban cluster of 10,000 to 49,999 persons and may include surrounding counties if there are strong economic ties between the counties, based on commuting patterns.

[4]Includes Asian, Native Hawaiian or Other Pacific Islander, American Indian or Alaska Native, and multiple races.

[5]General Educational Development credential given to persons who passed tests deemed equivalent to high school-level academic skills.

NOTES: Numbers may not add to totals and percent distributions may not add to 100% because of rounding, or because totals and percent distributions include a category of unknowns not reported in the table. Unknowns are included as a separate row in the table if the overall percentage is 5% or greater. For age, race, and sex, unknown responses were imputed, and less than 5% of responses were unknown. Percentages are based on unrounded numbers.

SOURCE: CDC/NCHS, National Home Health Aide Survey, 2007.

Table 2. Reasons for becoming a home health aide for currently employed home health aides, by age, sex, and race: United States, 2007

Reason	All home health aides	Under 25 years	25–34 years	35–44 years	45–54 years	55 years and over
	Number (standard error)					
All home health aides[1]	160,700 (11,479)	8,200 (1,789)	25,600 (3,285)	36,100 (3,378)	47,900 (4,775)	42,900 (5,061)
Home health aide jobs close to home	129,100 (9,929)	6,500 (1,664)	20,600 (2,836)	29,200 (3,078)	38,400 (4,073)	34,400 (4,663)
Want to eventually become a nurse	128,700 (10,210)	6,700 (1,678)	20,600 (3,126)	28,700 (2,873)	40,300 (4,551)	32,300 (4,192)
Provided care to friend or relative	123,200 (9,657)	5,000 (1,224)	20,800 (3,182)	27,200 (2,934)	38,100 (4,274)	32,100 (4,485)
Job was steady and secure	122,500 (8,709)	5,900 (1,401)	18,900 (2,539)	29,700 (3,150)	36,000 (3,790)	32,000 (3,636)
Thought it would give time to interact with patients or the elderly	121,900 (9,696)	6,700 (1,719)	19,800 (2,776)	28,300 (3,137)	36,700 (4,209)	30,400 (3,910)
Family member or friend was also one	119,200 (8,784)	6,600 (1,579)	21,000 (3,139)	27,000 (2,982)	33,900 (3,605)	30,600 (3,962)
Home health aide jobs available	102,600 (8,823)	4,200 (1,205)	16,300 (2,843)	23,200 (2,852)	31,000 (3,621)	28,000 (4,278)
Work hours fit schedule	98,800 (8,257)	4,900 (1,406)	16,900 (2,877)	21,800 (2,694)	31,100 (3,594)	24,200 (3,851)
Relative or friend receiving care	94,900 (7,359)	4,700 (1,197)	17,900 (3,015)	22,400 (2,692)	27,400 (3,214)	22,400 (3,265)
Like helping people	94,500 (8,065)	3,900 (1,053)	17,600 (2,537)	20,200 (2,612)	27,800 (3,610)	25,100 (3,886)
Prefer home care setting to facility	91,400 (7,778)	5,000 (1,292)	15,000 (2,136)	21,500 (2,752)	27,900 (3,709)	22,100 (3,229)
Wanted to work in health care	89,400 (6,671)	5,500 (1,334)	12,600 (1,831)	23,000 (2,659)	24,800 (2,912)	23,500 (3,640)
Other reason	66,700 (7,108)	†1,800 (769)	6,700 (1,449)	13,800 (2,167)	22,500 (3,443)	21,900 (3,682)
	Percent (standard error)					
Home health aide jobs close to home	80.3 (1.8)	79.4 (8.0)	80.6 (3.8)	80.7 (3.7)	80.1 (3.1)	80.3 (3.7)
Want to eventually become a nurse	80.0 (2.1)	81.6 (7.5)	80.5 (4.5)	79.4 (4.6)	84.2 (2.7)	75.4 (4.1)
Provided care to friend or relative	76.7 (1.7)	60.9 (8.7)	81.0 (4.0)	75.4 (4.2)	79.5 (3.0)	75.0 (3.9)
Job was steady and secure	76.2 (1.8)	71.7 (7.3)	74.0 (6.4)	82.1 (3.3)	75.1 (3.3)	74.7 (3.4)
Thought it would give time to interact with patients or the elderly	75.8 (1.9)	81.7 (6.6)	77.4 (4.7)	78.2 (3.7)	76.6 (3.3)	70.9 (4.3)
Family member or friend was also one	74.1 (2.0)	81.0 (8.0)	82.0 (3.7)	74.8 (3.9)	70.7 (3.9)	71.5 (4.6)
Home health aide jobs available	63.8 (2.3)	50.9 (9.6)	63.8 (6.3)	64.1 (4.7)	64.6 (3.5)	65.3 (4.5)
Work hours fit schedule	61.5 (2.0)	59.5 (11.0)	66.1 (5.3)	60.2 (5.1)	64.8 (3.8)	56.4 (4.6)
Relative or friend receiving care	59.0 (2.2)	57.2 (8.7)	70.0 (4.9)	62.0 (4.8)	57.2 (3.5)	52.3 (4.5)
Like helping people	58.8 (2.4)	47.3 (9.5)	68.5 (4.3)	55.9 (5.0)	58.0 (4.5)	58.6 (4.6)
Prefer home care setting to facility	56.9 (2.4)	60.6 (8.3)	58.4 (5.4)	59.4 (5.2)	58.2 (4.5)	51.6 (4.3)
Wanted to work in health care	55.6 (2.1)	67.1 (8.1)	49.1 (6.5)	63.6 (4.4)	51.6 (4.3)	54.9 (5.5)
Other reason	41.5 (2.9)	†22.2 (7.7)	26.1 (4.5)	38.2 (5.1)	46.9 (5.0)	51.1 (5.8)

See footnotes at end of table.

Table 2. Reasons for becoming a home health aide for currently employed home health aides, by age, sex, and race: United States, 2007—Con.

Reason	Female	Male	White	Black	Other[2]
	Number (standard error)				
All home health aides[1]	152,700 (11,032)	8,000 (1,607)	85,700 (7,623)	56,100 (6,889)	18,900 (3,514)
Home health aide jobs close to home	123,100 (9,436)	6,000 (1,457)	69,100 (6,495)	45,200 (6,200)	14,700 (2,779)
Want to eventually become a nurse	123,900 (10,035)	4,800 (1,179)	69,900 (6,843)	45,200 (5,781)	13,500 (3,010)
Provided care to friend or relative	117,300 (9,351)	5,900 (1,424)	66,300 (6,226)	41,500 (5,900)	15,300 (3,363)
Job was steady and secure	116,200 (8,256)	6,300 (1,457)	64,000 (5,971)	42,700 (5,508)	15,700 (3,303)
Thought it would give time to interact with patients or the elderly	115,700 (9,396)	6,200 (1,407)	63,700 (6,123)	43,900 (6,185)	14,300 (3,228)
Family member or friend was also one	112,000 (8,506)	7,200 (1,490)	62,700 (6,000)	42,700 (5,523)	13,800 (2,551)
Home health aide jobs available	97,200 (8,532)	5,500 (1,375)	52,300 (5,098)	37,600 (5,279)	12,800 (3,083)
Work hours fit schedule	94,100 (8,122)	4,800 (1,182)	51,200 (5,209)	37,900 (5,400)	9,700 (2,315)
Relative or friend receiving care	90,500 (7,104)	4,400 (1,184)	49,300 (5,063)	35,000 (5,059)	10,600 (2,896)
Like helping people	90,700 (7,928)	3,900 (1,086)	49,100 (5,128)	32,500 (4,789)	13,000 (3,188)
Prefer home care setting to facility	86,900 (7,700)	†4,500 (1,231)	45,700 (4,629)	33,600 (4,498)	12,100 (3,076)
Wanted to work in health care	85,300 (6,526)	4,100 (1,021)	45,700 (4,290)	31,800 (4,407)	11,900 (2,566)
Other reason	62,500 (6,778)	†4,200 (1,114)	35,300 (3,949)	21,600 (4,139)	9,800 (2,843)
	Percent (standard error)				
Home health aide jobs close to home	80.6 (1.8)	75.1 (8.3)	80.7 (2.2)	80.6 (3.4)	77.8 (6.5)
Want to eventually become a nurse	81.1 (2.1)	59.5 (10.6)	81.7 (2.3)	80.6 (3.2)	71.2 (7.9)
Provided care to friend or relative	76.8 (1.8)	74.0 (8.8)	77.4 (2.2)	74.0 (3.6)	81.1 (5.5)
Job was steady and secure	76.1 (1.8)	78.8 (7.9)	74.7 (2.9)	76.1 (4.0)	83.1 (5.3)
Thought it would give time to interact with patients or the elderly	75.7 (2.0)	77.4 (8.4)	74.3 (2.3)	78.3 (3.5)	75.4 (7.3)
Family member or friend was also one	73.3 (2.0)	90.0 (7.6)	73.2 (2.7)	76.0 (3.8)	72.7 (6.0)
Home health aide jobs available	63.6 (2.4)	68.3 (9.5)	61.0 (2.8)	67.0 (4.2)	67.4 (8.5)
Work hours fit schedule	61.6 (2.2)	59.5 (10.7)	59.8 (2.7)	67.6 (3.8)	51.2 (7.6)
Relative or friend receiving care	59.3 (2.2)	54.6 (10.5)	57.6 (2.9)	62.3 (3.7)	56.0 (8.8)
Like helping people	59.4 (2.5)	48.3 (10.4)	57.3 (3.1)	57.9 (4.4)	68.5 (7.8)
Prefer home care setting to facility	56.9 (2.6)	†55.8 (10.5)	53.4 (2.7)	59.8 (4.2)	64.0 (8.5)
Wanted to work in health care	55.8 (2.0)	50.8 (10.5)	53.3 (2.3)	56.6 (4.6)	62.8 (6.4)
Other reason	40.9 (2.8)	†52.9 (10.2)	41.2 (3.1)	38.6 (5.5)	51.7 (9.0)

† Estimate does not meet standards of reliability or precision because the sample size is between 30 and 59, or the sample size is greater than 59 but has a relative standard error of 30% or more.

[1]Includes home health aides currently employed by agencies that provide home health care services, hospice care services, or both types of services, and currently serve or recently served home health or hospice care patients. Agencies that provided only homemaker services or housekeeping services, assistance with instrumental activities of daily living, or durable medical equipment and supplies were excluded from the survey.

[2]Includes Asian, Native Hawaiian or Other Pacific Islander, American Indian or Alaska Native, and multiple races.

NOTES: For each reason, less than 5% of responses were unknown; in this table, these unknowns were treated as "no" responses. For age, race, and sex, unknown responses were imputed, and less than 5% of responses were unknown. Percentages are based on unrounded numbers.

SOURCE: CDC/NCHS, National Home Health Aide Survey, 2007.

Table 3. Employer and aide characteristics of currently employed home health aides, by whether they would become a home health aide again: United States, 2007

Characteristic	All home health aides		Definitely become one		Probably become one, probably or definitely not become one	
	Number (standard error)		Percent distribution (standard error)			
All home health aides[1]	160,700 (11,479)	100.0	72.2 (2.2)		27.8 (2.2)	
Employer characteristic						
Type of care provided:						
Home health care only	119200 (11,329)	100.0	71.7 (2.9)		28.2 (2.9)	
Hospice care only	20,000 (1,605)	100.0	75.9 (2.6)		24.1 (2.6)	
Home health and hospice care	21,500 (3,372)	100.0	71.3 (2.9)		28.7 (2.9)	
Ownership:						
Proprietary	101,700 (10,833)	100.0	70.2 (3.1)		29.8 (3.1)	
Voluntary nonprofit	51,400 (6,630)	100.0	76.0 (3.1)		24.0 (3.1)	
Government and other.	†7,600 †(2,417)	100.0	73.3 (3.5)		26.7 (3.5)	
Geographic region:						
Northeast.	23,600 (3,979)	100.0	73.3 (3.5)		26.7 (3.5)	
Midwest.	49,400 (7,529)	100.0	65.2 (4.8)		34.8 (4.8)	
South	75,600 (10,541)	100.0	77.2 (3.0)		22.8 (3.0)	
West.	12,100 (2,340)	100.0	67.3 (5.6)		32.7 (5.6)	
Location:						
Metropolitan statistical area[2]	135,000 (11,251)	100.0	72.6 (2.6)		27.4 (2.6)	
Micropolitan statistical area[3]	16,700 (2,120)	100.0	68.0 (3.1)		31.9 (3.1)	
Other location	9,000 (1,276)	100.0	74.0 (2.6)		26.0 (2.6)	
Chain affiliation:						
Part of a chain	48,100 (6,857)	100.0	69.8 (3.9)		30.1 (3.9)	
Not part of a chain	112,600 (11,014)	100.0	73.2 (2.7)		26.8 (2.7)	
Aide characteristic						
Age at time of interview:						
Under 25 years	8,200 (1,789)	100.0	49.9 (10.5)		†50.1 (10.5)	
25–34 years	25,600 (3,286)	100.0	69.4 (4.9)		30.6 (4.9)	
35–44 years	36,100 (3,379)	100.0	71.3 (4.5)		28.7 (4.5)	
45–54 years	47,900 (4,775)	100.0	76.3 (3.4)		23.7 (3.4)	
55 years and over	42,900 (5,062)	100.0	74.3 (4.5)		25.7 (4.5)	
Sex:						
Female	152,700 (11,032)	100.0	72.3 (2.2)		27.7 (2.2)	
Male.	8,000 (1,608)	100.0	70.9 (9.8)		†29.1 (9.8)	
Race:						
White	85,700 (7,624)	100.0	71.1 (3.1)		28.8 (3.1)	
Black	56,100 (6,889)	100.0	75.6 (3.6)		24.4 (3.6)	
Other[4]	18,900 (3,514)	100.0	67.0 (6.1)		33.0 (6.1)	
Hispanic or Latino origin:						
Hispanic or Latino	13,000 (2,717)	100.0	82.3 (5.8)		†17.7 (5.8)	
Not Hispanic or Latino.	144,900 (10,980)	100.0	71.1 (2.3)		28.9 (2.3)	
Education:						
No high school diploma or GED certificate[5].	11,500 (2,349)	100.0	86.7 (5.6)		*	*
GED certificate[5]	22,900 (3,258)	100.0	73.2 (5.6)		26.8 (5.6)	
High school diploma	60,600 (5,563)	100.0	74.4 (3.1)		25.6 (3.1)	
Some college or trade school	54,100 (5,004)	100.0	66.6 (3.7)		33.4 (3.7)	
College graduate or postgraduate.	9,400 (2,361)	100.0	69.0 (10.3)		†31.0 (10.3)	
Marital status:						
Married or living with partner.	80,800 (6,329)	100.0	70.7 (3.1)		29.3 (3.1)	
Widowed, divorced, or separated	51,400 (5,314)	100.0	77.6 (3.5)		22.4 (3.5)	
Never married.	26,300 (3,888)	100.0	65.8 (5.9)		34.2 (5.9)	
Citizenship:						
U.S. citizen.	151,300 (10,985)	100.0	71.8 (2.3)		28.2 (2.3)	
By birth	135,500 (10,586)	100.0	71.1 (2.3)		28.8 (2.3)	
By naturalization	15,800 (3,377)	100.0	77.3 (6.6)		†22.7 (6.6)	
Not U.S. citizen	7,200 (1,785)	100.0	78.8 (7.5)		*	*

See footnotes at end of table.

Table 3. Employer and aide characteristics of currently employed home health aides, by whether they would become a home health aide again: United States, 2007—Con.

Characteristic	All home health aides		Definitely become one		Probably become one, probably or definitely not become one	
	Number (standard error)		Percent distribution (standard error)			
Family income:						
Less than $20,000	34,500	(4,441)	100.0	68.2	(5.4)	31.8	(5.4)
$20,000–$29,999	40,800	(4,428)	100.0	75.8	(4.0)	24.1	(4.0)
$30,000–$39,999	32,900	(3,625)	100.0	73.0	(5.3)	27.0	(5.3)
$40,000–$49,999	17,300	(2,743)	100.0	75.3	(6.6)	24.7	(6.6)
$50,000 or more	26,700	(3,202)	100.0	70.9	(5.2)	29.1	(5.2)
Unknown	8,400	(2,000)	100.0	†65.7	(10.5)	†34.3	(10.5)

† Estimate does not meet standards of reliability or precision because the sample size is between 30 and 59, or the sample size is greater than 59 but has a relative standard error of 30% or more.

* Estimate does not meet standards of reliability or precision because the sample size is fewer than 30.

[1]Includes home health aides currently employed by agencies that provide home health care services, hospice care services, or both types of services, and currently serve or recently served home health or hospice care patients. Agencies that provided only homemaker services or housekeeping services, assistance with instrumental activities of daily living, or durable medical equipment and supplies were excluded from the survey.

[2]A county or group of contiguous counties that contains at least one urbanized area of 50,000 or more population and may contain other counties that are economically and socially integrated with the central county as measured by commuting.

[3]A nonmetropolitan county or group of contiguous nonmetropolitan counties that contains an urban cluster of 10,000 to 49,999 persons and may include surrounding counties if there are strong economic ties between the counties, based on commuting patterns.

[4]Includes Asian, Native Hawaiian or Other Pacific Islander, American Indian or Alaska Native, and multiple races.

[5]General Educational Development credential given to persons who passed tests deemed equivalent to high school-level academic skills.

NOTES: Numbers may not add to totals and percent distributions may not add to 100% because of rounding, or because totals and percent distributions include a category of unknowns not reported in the table. Unknowns are included as a separate row in the table if the overall percentage is 5% or greater. For age, race, and sex, unknown responses were imputed and less than 5% of responses were unknown. Percentages are based on unrounded numbers.

SOURCE: CDC/NCHS, National Home Health Aide Survey, 2007.

Table 4. Receipt of initial training and continuing education of currently employed home health aides, by employer and aide characteristics: United States, 2007

Characteristic	All home health aides				Received initial training				Took continuing education classes in the past 2 years			
	Number	Standard error	Percent distribution	Standard error	Number	Standard error	Percent	Standard error	Number	Standard error	Percent	Standard error
All home health aides[1]	160,700	(11,479)	100.0	...	134,900	(10,166)	83.9	(1.9)	146,300	(11,137)	91.0	(1.8)
Employer characteristic												
Type of care provided:												
Home health only	119,200	(11,329)	74.2	(2.6)	98,800	(9,979)	82.9	(2.5)	107,100	(10,950)	89.8	(2.4)
Hospice only	20,000	(1,605)	12.4	(1.3)	17,300	(1,465)	86.6	(1.9)	18,700	(1,583)	93.4	(1.3)
Home health and hospice	21,500	(3,372)	13.4	(2.2)	18,700	(3,071)	87.1	(3.0)	20,500	(3,314)	95.4	(2.0)
Ownership:												
Proprietary	101,700	(10,833)	63.3	(4.1)	84,800	(9,375)	83.3	(2.6)	89,300	(10,257)	87.8	(2.7)
Voluntary nonprofit, government, and other	59,000	(6,960)	36.7	(4.1)	50,100	(6,348)	84.9	(2.8)	57,000	(6,947)	96.5	(0.7)
Geographic region:												
Northeast	23,600	(3,979)	14.7	(2.6)	21,400	(3,732)	90.8	(2.8)	22,500	(3,951)	95.5	(1.7)
Midwest	49,400	(7,529)	30.8	(4.2)	39,900	(6,637)	80.7	(3.7)	44,100	(7,017)	89.2	(3.6)
South	75,600	(10,541)	47.0	(4.7)	63,800	(9,116)	84.5	(3.0)	69,600	(10,152)	92.1	(2.0)
West	12,100	(2,340)	7.5	(1.6)	9,700	(1,600)	80.2	(6.8)	10,000	(1,670)	82.8	(11.5)
Location of agency:												
Metropolitan statistical area[2]	135,000	(11,251)	84.0	(1.7)	113,600	(9,982)	84.1	(2.3)	124,000	(10,989)	91.8	(2.1)
Micropolitan statistical area[3]	16,700	(2,120)	10.4	(1.4)	13,500	(1,697)	80.7	(3.0)	14,400	(1,774)	85.9	(2.9)
Neither	9,000	(1,276)	5.6	(0.9)	7,800	(1,208)	86.8	(2.7)	7,900	(962)	88.1	(3.1)
Chain affiliation:												
Part of a chain	48,100	(6,857)	30.0	(4.0)	38,700	(5,463)	80.5	(3.8)	45,400	(6,719)	94.4	(1.7)
Not part of a chain	112,600	(11,014)	70.0	(4.0)	96,100	(9,935)	85.4	(2.2)	100,800	(10,496)	89.6	(2.4)
Aide characteristic												
Age at time of interview:												
Under 25 years	8,200	(1,789)	5.1	(1.1)	6,200	(1,596)	76.3	(7.8)	6,300	(1,575)	76.5	(8.2)
25–34 years	25,600	(3,286)	15.9	(1.8)	19,100	(2,832)	74.4	(4.9)	23,600	(3,215)	92.0	(3.2)
35–44 years	36,100	(3,379)	22.5	(1.8)	32,400	(3,345)	89.6	(2.5)	34,000	(3,348)	94.2	(2.3)
45–54 years	47,900	(4,775)	29.8	(2.0)	40,700	(4,189)	84.8	(3.4)	44,000	(4,627)	91.8	(2.7)
55 years and over	42,900	(5,062)	26.7	(2.0)	36,500	(4,567)	85.2	(3.7)	38,400	(4,692)	89.7	(4.1)
Sex:												
Female	152,700	(11,032)	95.0	(0.9)	128,100	(9,914)	83.9	(2.1)	138,800	(10,703)	90.9	(1.9)
Male	8,000	(1,608)	5.0	(0.9)	6,800	(1,474)	84.7	(7.8)	7,500	(1,565)	94.0	(3.0)
Race:												
White	85,700	(7,624)	53.3	(3.3)	67,700	(6,341)	79.1	(2.8)	76,600	(7,041)	89.4	(2.6)
Black	56,100	(6,889)	34.9	(3.4)	49,200	(6,120)	87.6	(3.0)	51,900	(6,743)	92.5	(2.5)
Other[4]	18,900	(3,514)	11.8	(1.9)	18,000	(3,457)	95.1	(2.4)	17,700	(3,480)	93.8	(2.9)
Hispanic or Latino origin:												
Hispanic or Latino	13,000	(2,717)	8.1	(1.7)	11,600	(2,525)	88.9	(4.8)	10,600	(2,160)	80.9	(7.0)
Not Hispanic or Latino	144,900	(10,980)	90.2	(1.8)	120,900	(9,678)	83.4	(2.1)	133,300	(10,646)	92.0	(1.7)
Education:												
No high school diploma or GED certificate[5]	11,500	(2,349)	7.1	(1.4)	11,000	(2,344)	96.1	(1.3)	10,000	(2,243)	86.8	(6.6)
GED certificate[5]	22,900	(3,258)	14.2	(1.7)	18,900	(2,998)	82.4	(5.8)	19,600	(2,737)	85.4	(4.8)
High school diploma	60,600	(5,563)	37.7	(2.4)	49,300	(5,207)	81.4	(3.6)	55,300	(5,512)	91.3	(2.5)
1–3 years of college or trade school	54,100	(5,004)	33.7	(1.9)	45,400	(4,515)	83.9	(3.3)	50,700	(4,809)	93.7	(1.8)
College graduate or post-graduate	9,400	(2,361)	5.9	(1.4)	8,400	(2,091)	88.8	(6.1)	8,900	(2,340)	94.0	(4.2)

See footnotes at end of table.

Table 4. Receipt of initial training and continuing education of currently employed home health aides, by employer and aide characteristics: United States, 2007—Con.

Characteristic	All home health aides				Received initial training				Took continuing education classes in the past 2 years			
	Number	Standard error	Percent distribution	Standard error	Number	Standard error	Percent	Standard error	Number	Standard error	Percent	Standard error
Marital status:												
Married or living with partner	80,800	(6,329)	50.3	(2.6)	67,400	(5,666)	83.4	(2.5)	74,600	(6,198)	92.3	(1.9)
Widowed, divorced, or separated	51,400	(5,314)	32.0	(2.3)	43,500	(4,840)	84.7	(3.4)	46,400	(4,887)	90.4	(3.5)
Never married	26,300	(3,888)	16.4	(2.0)	22,100	(3,628)	84.0	(3.8)	23,400	(3,803)	88.9	(3.7)
Citizenship:												
U.S. citizen	151,300	(10,985)	94.1	(1.3)	126,100	(9,637)	83.4	(2.0)	137,200	(10,590)	90.7	(1.9)
By birth	135,500	(10,586)	84.3	(2.4)	111,700	(9,230)	82.4	(2.2)	122,100	(10,062)	90.1	(2.0)
Naturalized	15,800	(3,377)	9.8	(2.0)	14,500	(2,836)	91.7	(4.3)	15,100	(3,370)	95.8	(2.3)
Not U.S. citizen	7,200	(1,785)	4.5	(1.1)	6,900	(1,780)	95.3	(2.8)	7,200	(1,785)	99.5	(0.3)
Family income:												
Less than $20,000	34,500	(4,441)	21.5	(2.2)	28,800	(3,672)	83.3	(4.3)	29,200	(4,126)	84.5	(3.8)
$20,000–$29,999	40,800	(4,428)	25.4	(2.1)	34,800	(3,827)	85.3	(3.6)	38,700	(4,388)	94.8	(1.3)
$30,000–$39,999	32,900	(3,625)	20.5	(1.7)	28,800	(3,396)	87.6	(3.5)	29,500	(3,416)	89.8	(4.4)
$40,000–$49,999	17,300	(2,743)	10.8	(1.5)	13,900	(2,577)	79.9	(5.5)	16,200	(2,692)	93.4	(3.8)
$50,000 or more	26,700	(3,202)	16.6	(1.8)	21,200	(2,695)	79.4	(4.3)	25,000	(3,136)	93.7	(2.5)
Unknown	8,400	(2,000)	5.2	(1.1)	7,400	(1,900)	87.8	(7.3)	7,600	(1,900)	90.5	(5.6)

. . . Category not applicable.

[1] Includes home health aides currently employed by agencies that provide home health care services, hospice care services, or both types of services, and currently serve or recently served home health or hospice care patients. Agencies that provided only homemaker services or housekeeping services, assistance with instrumental activities of daily living, or durable medical equipment and supplies were excluded from the survey.

[2] A county or group of contiguous counties that contains at least one urbanized area of 50,000 or more population and may contain other counties that are economically and socially integrated with the central county as measured by commuting.

[3] A nonmetropolitan county or group of contiguous nonmetropolitan counties that contains an urban cluster of 10,000 to 49,999 persons and may include surrounding counties if there are strong economic ties between the counties, based on commuting patterns.

[4] Includes Asian, Native Hawaiian or Other Pacific Islander, American Indian or Alaska Native, and multiple races.

[5] General Educational Development credential given to persons who passed tests deemed equivalent to high school-level academic skills.

NOTES: Numbers may not add to totals and percent distributions may not add to 100% because of rounding, or because totals and percent distributions include a category of unknowns not reported in the table. Unknowns are included as a separate row in the table if the overall percentage is 5% or greater. For age, race, and sex, unknown responses were imputed, and less than 5% of responses for were unknown. Percentages are based on the unrounded numbers.

SOURCE: CDC/NCHS, National Home Health Aide Survey, 2007.

Table 5. Assessment of initial training of currently employed home health aides, by employer, training, and aide characteristics: United States, 2007

Characteristic	Received initial training to become a home health aide					
	Number (standard error)			Percent distribution (standard error)		
	Total	Well prepared	Somewhat or not at all prepared	Total	Well prepared	Somewhat or not at all prepared
All home health aides[1]	134,900 (10,166)	110,800 (8,954)	24,000 (3,291)	100.0	82.2 (2.1)	17.8 (2.1)
Employer characteristic						
Type of care provided:						
Home health only	98,800 (9,979)	82,200 (8,806)	16,600 (3,165)	100.0	83.2 (2.8)	16.8 (2.8)
Hospice only	17,300 (1,465)	13,400 (1,137)	4,000 (646)	100.0	77.1 (2.8)	22.9 (2.8)
Home health and hospice	18,700 (3,071)	15,300 (2,719)	3,400 (707)	100.0	81.6 (3.2)	18.1 (3.2)
Ownership:						
Proprietary	84,800 (9,375)	71,800 (8,262)	12,900 (2,953)	100.0	84.7 (3.0)	15.3 (3.0)
Voluntary nonprofit, government, and other	50,100 (6,348)	39,000 (5,400)	11,100 (1,700)	100.0	77.8 (2.6)	22.1 (2.6)
Geographic region:						
Northeast	21,400 (3,732)	17,800 (3,363)	3,500 (829)	100.0	83.3 (3.4)	16.4 (3.4)
Midwest	39,900 (6,637)	31,400 (5,642)	8,500 (2,003)	100.0	78.7 (4.0)	21.3 (4.0)
South	63,800 (9,116)	53,400 (7,972)	10,400 (2,648)	100.0	83.7 (3.5)	16.3 (3.5)
West	9,700 (1,600)	8,200 (1,434)	1,600 (346)	100.0	83.8 (3.0)	16.2 (3.0)
Location of agency:						
Metropolitan statistical area[2]	113,600 (9,982)	94,000 (8,793)	19,600 (3,253)	100.0	82.7 (2.5)	17.2 (2.5)
Micropolitan statistical area[3]	13,500 (1,697)	11,000 (1,600)	2,500 (308)	100.0	81.8 (2.5)	18.2 (2.5)
Other location	7,800 (1,208)	5,800 (871)	2,000 (411)	100.0	74.5 (2.6)	25.5 (2.6)
Chain affiliation:						
Part of a chain	38,700 (5,463)	31,900 (4,827)	6,800 (1,429)	100.0	82.4 (3.1)	17.6 (3.1)
Not part of a chain	96,100 (9,935)	78,900 (8,643)	17,200 (3,072)	100.0	82.1 (2.7)	17.9 (2.7)
Training characteristic						
Type of classroom or formal training to become a home health aide:						
Mostly hands-on	20,600 (3,018)	16,800 (2,891)	3,800 (976)	100.0	81.6 (4.7)	18.4 (4.7)
Mostly classroom study	21,500 (2,766)	13,000 (2,096)	8,400 (1,715)	100.0	60.7 (6.1)	39.0 (6.1)
Evenly split between hands-on and classroom study	92,800 (7,849)	81,000 (7,184)	11,800 (1,892)	100.0	87.2 (1.8)	12.8 (1.8)
Initial training location:						
Home health or hospice agency	38,100 (4,342)	32,500 (4,056)	5,600 (1,292)	100.0	85.3 (3.2)	14.6 (3.2)
Nursing facility, hospital, or other health facility	24,100 (3,192)	20,400 (3,121)	3,700 (691)	100.0	84.5 (3.2)	15.5 (3.2)
High school or vocational, or technical school or community college, or other[4]	72,700 (7,000)	58,000 (6,000)	14,700 (2,852)	100.0	80.0 (3.3)	20.2 (3.3)
Aide characteristic						
Become an aide again:						
Definitely become one	98,900 (8,491)	83,900 (7,752)	15,000 (2,060)	100.0	84.8 (1.9)	15.2 (1.9)
Probably become one	28,600 (3,255)	21,000 (2,624)	7,600 (1,857)	100.0	73.5 (5.3)	26.5 (5.3)
Probably or definitely not become one	7,400 (2,101)	†5,900 (2,056)	†1,400 (510)	100.0	†80.0 (8.0)	†19.3 (7.9)

† Estimate does not meet standards of reliability or precision because the sample size is between 30 and 59, or the sample size is greater than 59 but has a relative standard error of 30% or more.

[1] Includes home health aides currently employed by agencies that provide home health care services, hospice care services, or both types of services, and currently serve or recently served home health or hospice care patients. Agencies that provided only homemaker services or housekeeping services, assistance with instrumental activities of daily living, or durable medical equipment and supplies were excluded from the survey.

[2] A county or group of contiguous counties that contains at least one urbanized area of 50,000 or more population and may contain other counties that are economically and socially integrated with the central county as measured by commuting.

[3] A nonmetropolitan county or group of contiguous nonmetropolitan counties that contains an urban cluster of 10,000 to 49,999 persons and may include surrounding counties if there are strong economic ties between the counties, based on commuting patterns.

[4] Other includes Red Cross training and training outside the United States or county or state health departments.

SOURCE: CDC/NCHS, National Home Health Aide Survey, 2007.

Table 6. Usefulness of continuing education for currently employed home health aides, by employer and training characteristics: United States, 2007

Characteristic	Took continuing education classes in the past 2 years					
	Number (standard error)			Percent distribution (standard error)		
	Total	Very useful	Somewhat or not at all useful	Total	Very useful	Somewhat or not at all useful
All home health aides[1]	146,300 (11,137)	115,800 (9,385)	30,500 (4,072)	100.0	79.1 (2.3)	20.9 (2.3)
Employer characteristic						
Type of care provided:						
Home health only	107,100 (10,950)	84,900 (9,259)	22,200 (3,939)	100.0	79.3 (3.0)	20.7 (3.0)
Hospice only	18,700 (1,583)	15,500 (1,368)	3,200 (490)	100.0	82.8 (2.2)	17.2 (2.2)
Home health and hospice	20,500 (3,314)	15,400 (2,461)	5,100 (1,150)	100.0	75.0 (3.3)	25.0 (3.3)
Ownership:						
Proprietary	89,300 (10,257)	70,200 (8,441)	19,100 (3,724)	100.0	78.6 (3.3)	21.4 (3.3)
Voluntary nonprofit, government, and other	57,000 (6,947)	45,600 (6,066)	11,400 (1,901)	100.0	79.9 (2.8)	20.1 (2.8)
Geographic region:						
Northeast	22,500 (3,951)	18,400 (3,304)	4,200 (1,106)	100.0	81.5 (3.6)	18.5 (3.6)
Midwest	44,100 (7,017)	30,800 (5,538)	13,300 (3,049)	100.0	69.9 (5.3)	30.1 (5.3)
South	69,600 (10,152)	59,100 (8,624)	10,500 (2,734)	100.0	84.9 (3.0)	15.1 (3.0)
West	10,000 (1,670)	7,500 (1,367)	2,600 (583)	100.0	74.5 (4.5)	25.5 (4.5)
Location of agency:						
Metropolitan statistical area[2]	124,000 (10,989)	99,000 (9,303)	25,000 (3,973)	100.0	79.8 (2.6)	20.2 (2.6)
Micropolitan statistical area[3]	14,400 (1,774)	10,800 (1,229)	3,600 (804)	100.0	75.1 (3.6)	24.9 (3.6)
Neither	7,900 (962)	6,000 (706)	1,900 (434)	100.0	76.1 (3.9)	23.9 (3.9)
Chain affiliation:						
Part of a chain	45,400 (6,719)	34,400 (5,458)	11,100 (2,575)	100.0	75.7 (4.4)	24.3 (4.4)
Not part of a chain	100,800 (10,496)	81,400 (8,839)	19,400 (3,349)	100.0	80.7 (2.6)	19.3 (2.6)
Training characteristic						
Type of initial training[4]:						
Mostly hands-on	19,000 (2,857)	14,800 (2,511)	4,300 (1,201)	100.0	77.7 (5.5)	22.3 (5.5)
Mostly classroom study	19,800 (2,578)	14,200 (2,099)	5,600 (1,465)	100.0	71.8 (6.1)	28.2 (6.1)
Evenly split between hands-on and classroom study	87,000 (7,617)	71,700 (6,832)	15,300 (2,344)	100.0	82.4 (2.4)	17.6 (2.4)
Initial training location[4]:						
Home health or hospice agency	36,200 (4,245)	27,500 (3,736)	8,700 (2,144)	100.0	75.9 (5.2)	24.1 (5.2)
Nursing facility, hospital or other health facility	21,200 (2,756)	17,500 (2,479)	3,700 (951)	100.0	82.7 (4.0)	17.3 (4.0)
High school, or vocational or technical school or community college, and other[5]	68,500 (6,918)	55,700 (5,915)	12,800 (2,123)	100.0	81.4 (2.5)	18.7 (2.5)
Become an aide again:						
Definitely become one	107,400 (9,067)	92,600 (8,380)	14,800 (2,052)	100.0	86.2 (1.8)	13.8 (1.8)
Probably become one	30,600 (3,381)	19,500 (2,363)	11,100 (2,442)	100.0	63.7 (5.8)	36.3 (5.8)
Probably or definitely not become one	8,300 (2,202)	†3,700 (1,228)	†4,600 (1,315)	100.0	†44.9 (7.7)	†55.1 (7.7)

† Estimate does not meet standards of reliability or precision because the sample size is between 30 and 59, or the sample size is greater than 59 but has a relative standard error of 30% or more.

[1] Includes home health aides currently employed by agencies that provide home health care services, hospice care services, or both types of services, and currently serve or recently served home health or hospice care patients. Agencies that provided only homemaker services or housekeeping services, assistance with instrumental activities of daily living, or durable medical equipment and supplies were excluded from the survey.

[2] A county or group of contiguous counties that contains at least one urbanized area of 50,000 or more population and may contain other counties that are economically and socially integrated with the central county as measured by commuting.

[3] A nonmetropolitan county or group of contiguous nonmetropolitan counties that contains an urban cluster of 10,000 to 49,999 persons and may include surrounding counties if there are strong economic ties between the counties, based on commuting patterns.

[4] Numbers do not add to total receiving continuing education because some aides did not receive initial training.

[5] Other includes Red Cross training and training outside the United States or county or state health departments.

NOTES: Numbers may not add to totals and percent distributions may not add to 100% because of rounding, or because totals and percent distributions include a category of unknowns not reported in the table. Unknowns accounted for less than 5% of responses for each category presented in this table. Percentages are based on unrounded numbers.

SOURCE: CDC/NCHS, National Home Health Aide Survey, 2007.

Table 7. Preference in hours worked of currently employed home health aides, by employer characteristics: United States, 2007

Characteristic	All home health aides	Preference in number of hours worked			
		Total	Hours worked about right	Would prefer more hours	Would prefer fewer hours
	Number (standard error)	Percent distribution (standard error)			
All home health aides[1]	160,700 (11,479)	100.0	69.6 (2.0)	26.2 (2.0)	†3.7 (1.1)
Type of care provided					
Home health care only	119,200 (11,329)	100.0	67.2 (2.6)	28.9 (2.6)	* *
Hospice care only	20,000 (1,605)	100.0	79.3 (2.2)	15.8 (1.9)	†4.1 (1.2)
Home health and hospice care	21,500 (3,372)	100.0	73.6 (3.4)	21.4 (3.4)	†4.7 (2.5)
Ownership					
Proprietary	101,700 (10,833)	100.0	65.3 (2.8)	29.8 (2.9)	†4.4 (1.7)
Voluntary nonprofit, government, and other	59,000 (6,960)	100.0	77.0 (2.3)	20.2 (2.3)	†2.5 (1.0)
Location					
Metropolitan statistical area[2].	135,000 (11,251)	100.0	68.9 (2.3)	26.6 (2.3)	†4.0 (1.3)
Micropolitan statistical area[3]	16,700 (2,120)	100.0	74.0 (3.6)	23.5 (3.3)	†2.0 (0.7)
Neither.	9,000 (1,276)	100.0	71.3 (2.4)	25.5 (2.4)	* *
Chain affiliation					
Part of a chain	48,100 (6,857)	100.0	69.7 (3.0)	27.3 (3.1)	* *
Not part of a chain.	112,600 (11,014)	100.0	69.5 (2.6)	25.8 (2.5)	†4.4 (1.5)

† Estimate does not meet standards of reliability or precision because the sample size is between 30 and 59, or the sample size is greater than 59 but has a relative standard error of 30% or more.

* Estimate does not meet standards of reliability or precision because the sample size is fewer than 30.

[1]Includes home health aides currently employed by agencies that provide home health care services, hospice care services, or both, and currently serve or recently served home health or hospice care patients. Agencies that provided only homemaker services or housekeeping services, assistance with instrumental activities of daily living, or durable medical equipment and supplies were excluded from the survey.

[2]A county or group of contiguous counties that contains at least one urbanized area of 50,000 or more population and may contain other counties that are economically and socially integraed with the central county as measured by commuting.

[3]A nonmetropolitan county or group of contiguous nonmetropolitan counties that contains an urban cluster of 10,000–49,999 persons and may include surrounding counties if strong economic ties exist between the counties, based on commuting patterns.

NOTES: Numbers may not add to totals and percent distributions may not add to 100% because of rounding, or because totals and percent distributions include a category of unknowns not reported in the table. Unknowns accounted for less than 5% of responses for each category presented in this table. Percentages are based on unrounded numbers.

SOURCE: CDC/NCHS, National Home Health Aide Survey, 2007.

Table 8. Adequacy of time to assist patients with activities of daily living of currently employed home health aides, by employer characteristics: United States, 2007

Characteristic	All home health aides		Time for ADL[1] assistance to patients											
			More than enough time				Enough time				Not enough time			
	Number	Standard error	Number	Standard error	Percent	Standard error	Number	Standard error	Percent	Standard error	Number	Standard error	Percent	Standard error
All home health aides[2]	160,700	11,479	65,800	6,467	40.9	2.4	84,400	6,742	52.5	2.5	7,800	1,779	4.8	1.1
Type of care provided														
Home health only	119,200	11,329	50,800	6,406	42.6	3.1	59,600	6,394	50.0	3.1	†6,500	1,769	†5.5	1.5
Hospice only	20,000	1,605	8,800	898	44.0	2.5	10,600	991	53.0	2.5	†500	133	†2.6	0.7
Home health and hospice	21,500	3,372	6,100	979	28.5	3.9	14,200	2,726	65.9	4.1	†700	185	†3.4	1.0
Ownership														
Proprietary	101,700	10,833	43,700	5,821	43.0	3.1	50,200	5,845	49.3	3.0	†5,700	1,659	†5.6	1.6
Voluntary nonprofit, government, and other	59,000	6,960	22,100	3,659	37.4	3.9	34,200	4,578	58.0	4.2	†2,100	673	†3.5	1.1
Location														
Metropolitan statistical area[3]	135,000	11,251	56,600	6,382	41.9	2.8	68,800	6,575	51.0	2.9	†7,100	1,772	5.2	1.3
Micropolitan statistical area[4]	16,700	2,120	6,300	967	37.9	3.1	9,600	1,341	57.6	3.0	†600	161	†3.4	0.9
Other location	9,000	1,276	2,800	484	31.6	2.6	6,000	883	66.5	2.6	*	*	*	*
Chain affiliation														
Part of a chain	48,100	6,857	17,400	2,824	36.1	3.0	27,300	4,346	56.7	4.3	†3,000	1,122	†6.3	2.1
Not part of a chain	112,600	11,014	48,400	6,289	43.0	3.1	57,100	6,045	50.7	3.0	†4,700	1,424	†4.2	1.3

† Estimate does not meet standards of reliability or precision because the sample size is between 30 and 59, or the sample size is greater than 59 but has a relative standard error of 30% or more.

* Estimate does not meet standards of reliability or precision because the sample size is fewer than 30.

[1]Activities of daily living include bathing, dressing, eating, transferring, and toileting.

[2]Includes home health aides currently employed by agencies that provide home health care services, hospice care services, or both, and currently serve or recently served home health or hospice care patients. Agencies that provided only homemaker services or housekeeping services, assistance with instrumental activities of daily living, or durable medical equipment and supplies were excluded from the survey.

[3]A county or group of contiguous counties that contains at least one urbanized area of 50,000 or more population and may contain other counties that are economically and socially integrated with the central county as measured by commuting.

[4]A nonmetropolitan county or group of contiguous nonmetropolitan counties that contains an urban cluster of 10,000–49,999 persons and may include surrounding counties if strong economic ties exist between the counties, based on commuting patterns.

NOTES: Numbers may not add to totals and percent distributions may not add to 100% because of rounding, or because totals and percent distributions include a category of unknowns not reported in the table. Unknowns accounted for less than 5% of responses for each category presented in this table. Percentages are based on unrounded numbers.

SOURCE: CDC/NCHS, National Home Health Aide Survey, 2007.

Table 9. Total time worked as a home health aide among currently employed home health aides, by employer and aide characteristics: United States, 2007

Characteristic	All home health aides	Total	Total time worked as home health aide		
			Fewer than 5 years	6–10 years	11 years or more
	Number (standard error)		Percent distribution (standard error)		
All home health aides[1]	160,700 (11,479)	100.0	29.6 (2.2)	20.4 (2.4)	50.0 (3.2)
Employer characteristic					
Type of care provided:					
Home health care only	119,200 (11,329)	100.0	30.4 (2.9)	19.9 (3.1)	49.6 (4.2)
Hospice care only	20,000 (1,605)	100.0	31.6 (2.5)	20.0 (2.3)	48.4 (2.8)
Home health and hospice care	21,500 (3,372)	100.0	22.9 (3.0)	23.5 (4.5)	53.6 (5.7)
Ownership:					
Proprietary	101,700 (10,833)	100.0	34.6 (2.9)	22.4 (3.3)	43.0 (4.2)
Voluntary nonprofit, government, and other	59,000 (6,960)	100.0	21.0 (2.7)	16.9 (3.1)	62.0 (3.9)
Location:					
Metropolitan statistical area[2]	135,000 (11,251)	100.0	27.7 (2.5)	20.5 (2.8)	51.9 (3.8)
Micropolitan statistical area[3]	16,700 (2,120)	100.0	42.8 (4.3)	21.5 (2.6)	35.6 (3.9)
Other location	9,000 (1,276)	100.0	33.7 (2.8)	17.7 (2.9)	48.6 (3.6)
Chain affiliation:					
Part of a chain	48,100 (6,857)	100.0	31.9 (3.9)	20.2 (3.9)	47.8 (5.4)
Not part of a chain	112,600 (11,014)	100.0	28.6 (2.6)	20.5 (3.0)	50.9 (4.0)
Aide characteristic					
Age at time of interview:					
Under 25 years	8,200 (1,789)	100.0	92.3 (5.3)	* *	* *
25–34 years	25,600 (3,286)	100.0	55.0 (4.6)	31.2 (4.9)	13.8 (3.7)
35–44 years	36,100 (3,379)	100.0	29.6 (5.2)	20.7 (3.8)	49.7 (5.2)
45–54 years	47,900 (4,775)	100.0	17.2 (3.2)	18.6 (3.8)	64.2 (5.1)
55 years and over	42,900 (5,062)	100.0	16.3 (4.3)	18.1 (4.1)	65.6 (5.2)
Race:					
White	85,700 (7,624)	100.0	31.5 (3.1)	22.0 (3.1)	46.5 (3.6)
Black	56,100 (6,889)	100.0	26.1 (4.0)	16.3 (3.4)	57.7 (5.3)
Other[4]	18,900 (3,514)	100.0	31.6 (7.6)	†25.5 (6.6)	42.9 (6.1)
Hispanic or Latino origin:					
Hispanic	13,000 (2,717)	100.0	34.7 (8.1)	†14.9 (5.1)	50.5 (9.8)
Not Hispanic	144,900 (10,980)	100.0	29.4 (2.4)	20.2 (2.5)	50.4 (3.4)
Education:					
No high school diploma or GED[5]	11,500 (2,349)	100.0	†13.1 (5.3)	†25.6 (7.9)	61.3 (8.8)
High school diploma	22,900 (3,258)	100.0	30.3 (6.7)	11.6 (3.2)	58.0 (7.1)
GED[5]	60,600 (5,563)	100.0	34.0 (3.6)	20.1 (3.3)	45.9 (4.6)
1–3 year college or trade school	54,100 (5,004)	100.0	27.9 (3.8)	19.7 (3.8)	52.4 (4.4)
College graduate or post graduate	9,400 (2,361)	100.0	†31.7 (11.5)	* *	†38.8 (11.6)
Marital status:					
Married or living with partner	80,800 (6,329)	100.0	31.7 (2.8)	18.8 (2.5)	49.5 (3.3)
Widowed, divorced, separated	51,400 (5,314)	100.0	19.4 (4.1)	19.6 (3.7)	60.9 (5.0)
Never married	26,300 (3,888)	100.0	43.7 (5.0)	22.6 (5.9)	33.7 (5.6)
Family income:					
Less than $20,000	34,500 (4,441)	100.0	41.2 (6.3)	22.0 (3.9)	36.7 (6.1)
$20,000–$29,999	40,800 (4,428)	100.0	21.7 (3.4)	22.0 (4.1)	56.3 (4.9)
$30,000–$39,999	32,900 (3,625)	100.0	27.6 (4.9)	20.1 (4.8)	52.3 (5.6)
$40,000–$49,999	17,300 (2,743)	100.0	37.0 (7.6)	†8.6 (2.9)	54.5 (8.0)
$50,000 or more	26,700 (3,202)	100.0	28.9 (5.1)	19.4 (5.2)	51.7 (6.1)
Unknown	8,400 (2,000)	100.0	* *	†(35.2) (12.4)	†50.4 (12.1)

* Estimate does not meet standards of reliability or precision because the sample size is fewer than 30.
† Estimate does not meet standards of reliability or precision because the sample size is between 30 and 59, or the sample size is greater than 59 but has a relative standard error of 30% or more.
[1]Includes home health aides currently employed by agencies that provide home health care services, hospice care services, or both, and currently serve or recently served home health or hospice care patients. Agencies that provided only homemaker services or housekeeping services, assistance with instrumental activities of daily living, or durable medical equipment and supplies were excluded from the survey.
[2]A county or group of contiguous counties that contains at least one urbanized area of 50,000 or more population and may also contain other counties that are economically and socially integrated with the central county as measured by commuting.
[3]A nonmetropolitan county or group of contiguous nonmetropolitan counties that contains an urban cluster of 10,000–49,999 persons and may include surrounding counties if strong economic ties exist between the counties, based on commuting patterns.
[4]Includes Asian, Native Hawaiian or Other Pacific Islander, American Indian or Alaska Native, and multiple races.
[5]General Educational Development credential given to persons who passed tests deemed equivalent to high school-level academic skills.

NOTES: Numbers may not add to totals and percent distributions may not add to 100% because of rounding, or because totals and percent distributions include a category of unknowns not reported in the table. Unknowns are included as a separate row in the table if the overall percentage is 5% or greater. For age, race and sex, unknown responses were imputed, and less than 5% of responses were unknown. Percentages are based on unrounded numbers.

SOURCE: CDC/NCHS, National Home Health Aide Survey, 2007.

Table 10. Reasons for continuing in current job for currently employed home health aides, by age, sex, and race: United States, 2007

Reason for continuing in current job	All home health aides	Under 25 years	25–34 years	35–44 years	45–54 years	55 years and over
	Number (standard error)					
All home health aides[1]	160,700 (11,479)	8,200 (1,789)	25,600 (3,286)	36,100 (3,379)	47,900 (4,775)	42,900 (5,062)
Agency/management environment						
Career advancement opportunities	125,600 (8,818)	7,300 (1,748)	18,400 (2,364)	27,800 (2,970)	39,400 (4,094)	32,600 (3,953)
Opportunity to work overtime	114,200 (9,015)	3,900 (1,018)	19,200 (2,889)	23,600 (2,705)	34,700 (3,650)	32,800 (4,076)
Flexible schedule or hours	109,700 (8,375)	5,400 (1,546)	18,400 (2,863)	26,400 (2,920)	32,900 (3,799)	26,800 (3,566)
Benefits	104,500 (7,904)	4,800 (1,363)	17,200 (2,728)	23,300 (2,692)	30,800 (3,675)	28,400 (3,811)
Professional/personal environment						
Enjoy working with other members of care team . .	110,500 (8,335)	3,400 (861)	19,600 (3,127)	26,000 (2,793)	29,700 (3,487)	31,800 (4,284)
Enjoy caring for others	105,100 (8,193)	4,400 (1,215)	17,000 (2,351)	24,200 (2,922)	32,600 (3,648)	26,900 (3,725)
Able to work independently	99,700 (7,798)	4,900 (1,416)	15,400 (2,860)	21,300 (2,529)	33,400 (3,923)	24,800 (3,440)
Feeling good about work environment	94,100 (7,043)	3,900 (1,051)	18,800 (3,055)	21,300 (2,543)	26,600 (3,009)	23,600 (3,530)
Enjoy working with supervisor	93,800 (7,041)	3,400 (1,010)	15,000 (2,436)	21,100 (2,631)	26,500 (2,948)	27,800 (3,747)
Other reasons	55,800 (5,858)	* *	9,100 (1,981)	11,500 (2,188)	17,300 (2,489)	7,800 (1,973)
Agency/management environment	Percent (standard error)					
Career advancement opportunities	78.1 (1.9)	89.4 (5.1)	71.7 (5.2)	77.0 (4.6)	82.3 (3.4)	76.0 (3.8)
Opportunity to work overtime	71.0 (2.5)	47.3 (8.6)	75.1 (4.6)	65.3 (5.0)	72.4 (4.4)	76.5 (4.1)
Flexible schedule or hours	68.3 (2.5)	65.6 (10.0)	71.7 (5.0)	72.9 (4.5)	68.6 (3.7)	62.5 (3.9)
Benefits	65.0 (2.3)	58.9 (10.3)	67.2 (5.2)	64.5 (4.5)	64.2 (5.1)	66.3 (4.7)
Professional/personal environment						
Enjoy working with other members of care team . .	68.8 (2.4)	41.3 (9.6)	76.5 (4.8)	72.0 (4.3)	62.0 (5.5)	74.2 (4.6)
Enjoy caring for others	65.4 (2.4)	54.2 (9.6)	66.5 (4.6)	66.9 (5.0)	67.9 (3.7)	62.8 (5.0)
Able to work independently	62.0 (2.7)	59.7 (10.1)	60.2 (6.4)	58.8 (4.6)	69.7 (3.8)	57.8 (5.6)
Feeling good about work environment	58.6 (2.5)	47.4 (8.6)	73.4 (5.0)	59.0 (5.2)	55.5 (3.4)	55.0 (5.9)
Enjoy working with supervisor	58.3 (2.3)	41.6 (9.2)	58.6 (5.1)	58.3 (5.4)	55.4 (3.7)	64.8 (4.5)
Other reasons	34.7 (2.7)	* *	35.4 (5.9)	31.7 (5.1)	36.0 (4.3)	37.3 (4.9)

Reason for continuing in current job	All home health aides	Female	Male	White	Black	Other[2]
	Number (standard error)					
All home health aides[1]	160,700 (11,479)	152,700 (11,032)	8,000 (1,608)	85,700 (7,624)	56,100 (6,889)	18,900 (3,514)
Agency/management environment						
Career advancement opportunities	125,600 (8,818)	120,300 (8,549)	5,200 (1,193)	68,400 (6,116)	43,100 (5,373)	14,100 (2,649)
Opportunity to work overtime	114,200 (9,015)	107,400 (8,454)	6,700 (1,534)	62,100 (6,088)	41,500 (5,604)	10,600 (2,243)
Flexible schedule or hours	109,700 (8,375)	104,400 (8,050)	5,400 (1,291)	60,500 (6,247)	36,000 (5,038)	13,200 (2,355)
Benefits	104,500 (7,904)	98,900 (7,434)	5,600 (1,360)	53,800 (4,843)	38,500 (5,948)	12,200 (2,339)
Professional/personal environment						
Enjoy working with other members of care team . .	110,500 (8,335)	104,300 (7,883)	6,300 (1,508)	60,700 (5,838)	38,400 (5,581)	11,400 (2,292)
Enjoy caring for others	105,100 (8,193)	100,300 (7,794)	4,800 (1,197)	51,800 (4,820)	39,700 (5,631)	13,600 (2,561)
Able to work independently	99,700 (7,798)	94,200 (7,482)	5,500 (1,269)	53,400 (5,215)	33,400 (4,949)	12,900 (2,431)
Feeling good about work environment	94,100 (7,043)	89,600 (6,764)	4,500 (1,129)	52,100 (5,172)	34,900 (5,242)	7,100 (1,569)
Enjoy working with supervisor	93,800 (7,041)	87,800 (6,796)	6,000 (1,430)	53,200 (5,469)	30,300 (4,656)	10,200 (2,172)
Other reasons	55,800 (5,858)	51,900 (5,388)	†3,900 (1,221)	31,900 (4,091)	16,100 (3,380)	7,800 (1,973)
Agency/management environment	Percent (standard error)					
Career advancement opportunities	78.1 (1.9)	78.8 (1.9)	65.5 (10.8)	79.8 (2.6)	76.7 (3.2)	74.5 (6.0)
Opportunity to work overtime	71.0 (2.5)	70.3 (2.5)	84.4 (5.4)	72.4 (3.0)	73.9 (4.3)	56.2 (7.7)
Flexible schedule or hours	68.3 (2.5)	68.3 (2.4)	67.1 (10.2)	70.6 (3.1)	64.1 (4.0)	70.0 (9.5)
Benefits	65.0 (2.3)	64.8 (2.3)	70.4 (9.3)	62.8 (2.9)	68.6 (4.2)	64.6 (6.3)
Professional/personal environment						
Enjoy working with other members of care team . .	68.8 (2.4)	68.3 (2.5)	78.3 (7.2)	70.9 (2.6)	68.4 (4.3)	60.4 (6.2)
Enjoy caring for others	65.4 (2.4)	65.7 (2.4)	60.0 (10.2)	60.4 (3.1)	70.7 (4.3)	72.1 (6.4)
Able to work independently	62.0 (2.7)	61.7 (2.8)	68.7 (10.1)	62.4 (2.8)	59.5 (4.6)	68.1 (9.7)
Feeling good about work environment	58.6 (2.5)	58.7 (2.6)	56.6 (10.3)	60.8 (3.0)	62.2 (4.4)	37.8 (8.3)
Enjoy working with supervisor	58.3 (2.3)	57.5 (2.4)	74.5 (8.8)	62.1 (3.1)	54.0 (4.5)	54.1 (9.3)
Other reasons	34.7 (2.7)	33.9 (2.6)	†49.0 (10.3)	37.2 (3.1)	28.6 (4.4)	41.3 (8.7)

* Estimate does not meet standards of reliability or precision.

† Estimate does not meet standards of reliability or precision because the sample size is between 30 and 59, or the sample size is greater than 59 but has a relative standard error of 30% or more.

[1] Includes home health aides currently employed by agencies that provide home health care services, hospice care services, or both, and currently serve or recently served home health or hospice care patients. Agencies that provided only homemaker services or housekeeping services, assistance with instrumental activities of daily living, or durable medical equipment and supplies were excluded from the survey.

[2] Includes Asian, Native Hawaiian or other Pacific Islander, American Indian or Alaska Native, and multiple races.

NOTES: For each reason for continuing in current job, less than 5% of responses were unknown; in this table, these unknowns were treated as no responses. For age, race, and sex, unknown responses were imputed, and less than 5% of responses were unknown. Percentages are based on unrounded numbers.

SOURCE: CDC/NCHS, National Home Health Aide Survey, 2007.

Table 11. Attitudes toward job, by overall job satisfaction of currently employed home health aides: United States, 2007

Job satisfaction	All home health aides[1]				Overall job satisfaction					
	Number (standard error)		Percent (standard error)		Extremely satisfied		Somewhat satisfied		Somewhat or extremely dissatisfied	
					Percent distribution (standard error)					
All home health aides[1]	160,700	(11,479)	100.0	. . .	46.7	(2.3)	40.4	(2.2)	11.7	(1.8)
Satisfaction with aspects of current job										
Doing challenging work:										
Extremely satisfied	95,000	(7,650)	59.1	(2.5)	77.0	(3.1)	45.9	(3.7)	38.8	(8.7)
Somewhat satisfied.	59,400n	(5,570)	37.0	(2.3)	22.2	(3.1)	51.5	(3.8)	49.2	(8.9)
Somewhat or extremely dissatisfied	†3,600	†(1,130)	†2.2	(0.7)	*	*	*	*	*	*
Benefits:										
Extremely satisfied	45,800	(4,488)	28.5	(2.4)	47.0	(3.3)	15.2	(2.5)	†3.9	(1.1)
Somewhat satisfied.	46,400	(4,580)	28.9	(2.4)	29.0	(3.0)	33.0	(3.6)	16.9	(4.6)
Somewhat or extremely dissatisfied	60,800	(7,164)	37.8	(2.9)	20.6	(2.7)	47.2	(4.1)	77.4	(5.3)
Salary:										
Extremely satisfied	27,700	(3,024)	17.2	(1.9)	31.6	(3.2)	5.2	(1.4)	*	*
Somewhat satisfied.	70,400	(5,943)	43.8	(2.6)	49.5	(3.2)	43.5	(3.6)	†26.4	(7.8)
Somewhat or extremely dissatisfied	60,800	(7,185)	37.8	(2.9)	18.8	(2.8)	51.3	(3.8)	70.7	(8.0)
Learning new skills:										
Extremely satisfied	90,100	(7,687)	56.0	(3.2)	73.0	(3.2)	46.7	(3.7)	25.9	(6.8)
Somewhat satisfied.	59,200	(6,363)	36.8	(2.7)	25.1	(3.1)	46.5	(3.7)	54.1	(8.5)
Somewhat or extremely dissatisfied	9,300	(1,881)	5.8	(1.1)	†1.5	(0.8)	6.7	(1.7)	†20.0	(6.4)
Perceived respect and value of work										
Society values or appreciates aides' work:										
Very much	90,200	(7,133)	56.1	(2.3)	62.5	(3.2)	52.2	(3.8)	50.0	(6.2)
Somewhat or not at all	67,600	(5,981)	42.0	(2.2)	37.3	(3.2)	46.4	(3.8)	50.0	(6.2)
Organization values or appreciates work aides do:										
Very much	106,600	(8,582)	66.3	(2.5)	89.0	(1.9)	51.2	(3.8)	34.6	(7.5)
Somewhat or not at all	51,600	(5,144)	32.1	(2.4)	10.8	(1.9)	48.0	(3.8)	65.2	(7.5)
Supervisor values or appreciates work aides do:										
Very much	122,900	(9,814)	76.5	(2.2)	94.3	(1.2)	66.5	(3.7)	46.7	(9.1)
Somewhat or not at all	34,100	(3,670)	21.2	(2.1)	5.6	(1.2)	30.6	(3.4)	53.1	(9.1)
Self-rated importance of aides' work:										
Very important.	155,100	(10,930)	96.5	(1.0)	99.6	(0.2)	96.7	(1.2)	92.8	(3.8)
Somewhat or not at all important	3,400	(1,013)	2.1	(0.6)	*	*	†2.7	(1.1)	*	*
Supervisor respects aide as part of health care team:										
A great deal	121,600	(9,651)	75.7	(2.1)	92.6	(2.1)	66.4	(3.1)	47.4	(8.7)
Somewhat or not at all	36,300	(3,745)	22.6	(2.1)	6.6	(1.5)	33.0	(3.1)	52.4	(8.6)
Patients respect aide as part of health care team:										
A great deal	144,000	(10,159)	89.6	(1.3)	91.7	(1.9)	89.9	(2.0)	88.8	(3.6)
Somewhat or not at all	12,300	(1,977)	7.6	(1.2)	5.5	(1.4)	9.7	(2.0)	†9.8	(3.4)
Commitment to field and job										
Become a home health aide again:										
Definitely yes	116,000	(9,281)	72.2	(2.2)	84.2	(2.1)	67.3	(3.2)	40.8	(7.0)
Probably yes.	34,500	(3,669)	21.5	(1.9)	14.7	(2.0)	25.7	(2.8)	34.2	(6.5)
Probably or definitely not	10,100	(2,332)	6.3	(1.4)	*	*	7.0	(2.0)	†25.0	(6.8)
Take current job again:										
Definitely yes	86,800	(6,853)	54.0	(2.3)	80.5	(3.0)	37.9	(3.6)	†8.3	(3.4)
Probably yes.	49,000	(4,758)	30.5	(2.0)	15.9	(2.7)	47.6	(3.4)	26.5	(5.8)
Probably or definitely not	22,500	(3,274)	14.0	(1.6)	*	*	14.2	(2.5)	58.7	(5.8)

. . . Category not applicable.

† Estimate does not meet standards of reliability or precision because the sample size is between 30 and 59, or the sample size is greater than 59 but has a relative standard error of 30% or more.

* Estimate does not meet standards of reliability or precision because the sample size is fewer than 30.

[1] Includes home health aides currently employed by agencies that provide home health care services, hospice care services, or both, and currently serve or recently served home health or hospice care patients. Agencies that provided only homemaker services or housekeeping services, assistance with instrumental activities of daily living, or durable medical equipment and supplies were excluded from the survey.

NOTES: Numbers may not add to totals and percent distributions may not add to 100% because of rounding, or because totals and percent distributions include a category of unknowns not reported in the table. Unknowns accounted for less than 5% of responses for each category presented in this table. Percentages are based on unrounded numbers.

SOURCE: CDC/NCHS, National Home Health Aide Survey, 2007.

Table 12. Mean and median hourly rate of pay for currently employed home health aides, by total length of time worked as a home health aide and employer characteristics: United States, 2007

Characteristic	All home health aides[1]		Total time worked as a home health aide						Percent (SE) of aides who received a pay increase in past 12 months
			5 years or fewer		6–10 years		More than 10 years		
	Mean hourly pay rate	Median hourly pay rate	Mean hourly pay rate	Median hourly pay rate	Mean hourly pay rate	Median hourly pay rate	Mean hourly pay rate	Median hourly pay rate	
	In dollars (SE)								
All home health aides[2]	$10.88 (0.45)	$10.51 (0.34)	$10.14 (0.75)	$9.99 (0.33)	$10.77 (0.65)	$10.00 (0.38)	$11.37 (0.70)	$11.85 (0.32)	56.7 (3.3)
Agency type and size[3]									
Home health only	10.83 (0.60)	10.00 (0.39)	10.04 (0.97)	9.45 (0.38)	10.74 (0.89)	9.49 (0.54)	11.35 (0.93)	11.50 (0.54)	51.6 (4.3)
Small	10.47 (1.31)	9.99 (1.96)	†10.04 (2.04)	†8.9 (1.06)	*	*	†8.97 (3.23)	11.66 (2.29)	41.5 (8.7)
Medium	10.35 (1.15)	9.41 (0.47)	8.97 (0.56)	8.91 (0.36)	†10.43 (1.85)	†9.41 (0.36)	11.22 (2.22)	10.11 (0.92)	54.4 (8.4)
Large	11.60 (0.79)	11.18 (0.58)	11.93 (2.05)	10.52 (0.64)	10.04 (0.59)	10.00 (0.63)	11.89 (0.81)	12.15 (0.66)	55.4 (5.5)
Hospice only	11.13 (0.30)	11.75 (0.28)	10.62 (0.50)	11.26 (0.44)	11.26 (0.39)	11.58 (0.47)	11.41 (0.51)	12.18 (0.33)	69.6 (2.8)
Small	10.04 (0.68)	10.96 (0.81)	10.15 (0.75)	9.96 (0.90)	†10.13 (1.79)	†9.77 (- - -)	9.81 (2.55)	12.41 (1.27)	47.0 (9.1)
Medium	11.38 (0.72)	11.64 (0.96)	10.48 (1.02)	10.07 (0.73)	11.05 (0.83)	11.53 (0.73)	11.83 (1.13)	12.82 (0.89)	65.5 (6.8)
Large	11.28 (0.34)	11.84 (0.28)	10.71 (0.69)	11.42 (0.42)	11.41 (0.43)	11.49 (0.51)	11.65 (0.49)	12.06 (0.29)	74.5 (2.9)
Home health and hospice	10.97 (0.53)	11.46 (0.53)	10.2 (0.41)	10.34 (0.36)	10.52 (0.40)	10.48 (0.46)	11.49 (0.90)	12.64 (0.58)	73.3 (5.3)
Small	8.15 (1.21)	9.99 (0.43)	9.19 (1.00)	9.91 (0.47)	†9.88 (0.71)	†9.69 (1.06)	†6.59 (2.39)	10.39 (1.09)	62.2 (9.3)
Medium	11.80 (0.78)	11.86 (0.80)	10.61 (0.74)	10.36 (0.84)	10.20 (1.24)	10.73 (0.77)	12.91 (0.77)	13.01 (1.09)	78.5 (7.2)
Large	10.13 (0.76)	10.49 (0.46)	8.20 (1.99)	10.04 (0.42)	10.61 (0.34)	10.47 (0.45)	10.89 (0.95)	11.74 (0.71)	69.0 (8.5)
Ownership									
Proprietary	10.28 (0.65)	9.49 (0.29)	10.04 (1.00)	9.00 (0.35)	10.70 (0.91)	9.48 (0.57)	10.25 (1.14)	10.00 (0.70)	44.9 (4.6)
Voluntary nonprofit	12.01 (0.46)	12.08 (0.28)	10.36 (0.37)	10.75 (0.21)	10.91 (0.48)	11.78 (0.47)	12.80 (0.63)	12.65 (0.40)	78.4 (3.7)
Government and other	11.32 (0.82)	10.50 (0.84)	10.64 (0.75)	10.34 (0.46)	10.95 (0.37)	10.42 (- - -)	11.92 (1.27)	12.62 (0.99)	68.1 (10.5)
Geographic region									
Northeast	10.42 (0.72)	11.12 (0.48)	8.10 (1.76)	10.35 (0.45)	10.53 (0.82)	10.89 (0.32)	11.61 (0.74)	12.49 (0.62)	62.2 (6.9)
Midwest	10.97 (0.74)	10.37 (0.40)	11.81 (1.78)	9.96 (0.43)	10.01 (0.72)	9.50 (0.79)	10.88 (0.63)	11.05 (0.53)	59.0 (6.3)
South	10.97 (0.77)	10.16 (0.67)	9.91 (0.70)	8.90 (0.50)	11.31 (1.21)	9.49 (0.90)	11.43 (1.38)	11.60 (0.70)	53.2 (5.2)
West	10.87 (1.26)	12.25 (0.77)	8.76 (1.96)	10.00 (0.97)	11.06 (1.15)	12.33 (0.47)	12.66 (1.36)	13.78 (1.04)	59.1 (5.5)
Location									
Metropolitan statistical area[4]	10.91 (0.44)	10.98 (0.48)	10.48 (0.95)	10.00 (0.37)	10.99 (0.76)	10.34 (0.54)	11.11 (0.56)	11.99 (0.42)	56.2 (3.8)
Micropolitan statistical area[5]	12.16 (2.41)	9.54 (0.26)	9.05 (0.30)	8.99 (0.24)	9.58 (0.49)	9.58 (0.50)	†17.46 (6.61)	10.73 (0.38)	56.4 (4.4)
Other location	8.12 (0.85)	9.17 (0.58)	8.44 (0.65)	7.96 (0.45)	9.54 (0.53)	9.71 (0.25)	7.38 (1.50)	9.36 (0.81)	64.8 (3.8)
Chain affiliation									
Part of a chain	10.33 (1.05)	10.00 (0.41)	9.34 (0.95)	9.82 (0.42)	10.36 (1.63)	9.48 (0.51)	10.98 (1.94)	10.95 (0.53)	47.5 (5.0)
Not part of a chain	11.12 (0.46)	10.99 (0.49)	10.52 (1.00)	9.99 (0.33)	10.94 (0.62)	10.49 (0.67)	11.53 (0.59)	12.00 (0.48)	60.7 (4.1)

† Estimate does not meet standards of reliability or precision because the sample size is between 30 and 59, or the sample size is greater than 59 but has a relative standard error of 30% or more.

* Estimate does not meet standards of reliability or precision because the sample size is fewer than 30.

- - - Data not available.

[1]Includes aides for whom time worked as a home health aide was unknown.

[2]Includes home health aides currently employed by agencies that provide home health care services, hospice care services, or both, and currently serve or recently served home health or hospice care patients. Agencies that provided only homemaker services or housekeeping services, assistance with instrumental activities of daily living, or durable medical equipment and supplies were excluded from the survey.

[3]Provider size is based on agency type. For home health care agencies, small was fewer than 47 current patients, medium was 47–105, and large was 106 or more. For hospice care agencies, small was 28 or fewer current patients, medium was 29–72, and large was 72 or more. For providers of both home health and hospice care, small was 79 or fewer current patients (both hospice and home health care), medium was 80–224, and large was 225 or more.

[4]A county or group of contiguous counties that contains at least one urbanized area of 50,000 or more population and may contain other counties that are economically and socially integrated with the central county as measured by commuting.

[5]A nonmetropolitan county or group of contiguous nonmetropolitan counties that contains an urban cluster of 10,000 to 49,999 persons and may include surrounding counties if there are strong economic ties between the counties, based on commuting patterns.

NOTES: Unknowns were excluded when calculating mean and median hourly pay. Among home health aides, 6.67% were missing some information necessary to calculate hourly pay rate. SE is standard error.

SOURCE: CDC/NCHS, National Home Health Aide Survey, 2007.

Table 13. Percentage of currently employed home health aides reporting benefits offered by employer, by employer size and type: United States, 2007

Employee benefits	All agencies		Home health only				Hospice only				Home health and hospice			
	Benefit offered[2]	Unknown	Total	Small	Medium	Large	Total	Small	Medium	Large	Total	Small	Medium	Large
							Percent							
All home health aides[3]	100.0	100.0	100.0	100.0	100.0	100.0	100.0	100.0	100.0	100.0	100.0	100.0	100.0	100.0
Health insurance coverage	72.7	†3.0	66.0	43.0	59.3	79.0	94.3	83.1	97.0	95.5	89.2	71.4	87.7	91.1
Extra pay for working holidays	62.0	4.3	59.6	53.3	44.1	73.0	65.2	54.2	56.2	70.4	72.1	70.5	65.4	75.1
Paid time off, such as vacation or personal days[4]	59.1	†3.3	51.5	25.6	56.4	56.7	86.1	66.0	91.8	87.3	76.0	73.1	70.1	75.8
Dental, vision, or drug benefits	56.0	7.0	46.3	23.6	32.7	66.3	87.6	66.2	86.1	90.8	80.3	55.9	74.3	85.6
Disability and/or life insurance	53.2	10.2	45.2	31.2	32.1	60.7	83.5	45.7	89.7	87.6	69.7	57.7	66.2	68.9
Paid holidays off	51.2	†2.8	42.9	†16.4	41.0	54.4	87.3	60.2	91.8	89.5	63.8	55.2	64.0	60.0
Paid sick leave	50.5	4.8	41.5	†22.6	33.0	55.4	82.8	64.9	87.4	85.1	70.6	57.8	68.9	69.0
Retirement or pension plan	49.2	10.6	40.4	†7.8	26.9	63.1	78.2	55.1	75.8	83.5	71.3	59.8	67.2	72.2
Bonuses	36.8	4.5	36.1	†26.1	24.3	48.4	37.8	29.8	43.8	38.5	39.3	35.6	28.8	40.7
Tuition	30.4	12.9	24.5	†14.6	†17.6	33.3	50.0	†21.2	48.5	55.1	44.8	38.8	35.6	47.9
Cell phone for work	24.3	†1.9	18.2	*	†7.0	34.0	49.9	22.0	43.9	55.4	34.0	36.1	20.8	36.7
Time off for good work	8.8	5.5	8.1	*	*	†11.7	16.8	*	†9.0	20.1	5.6	*	†6.5	†5.9
Paid child care assistance	6.1	14.5	5.2	*	*	†9.1	7.8	*	*	†7.9	9.5	*	†4.4	†12.7
Other benefits	14.6	*	12.4	*	†9.0	19.2	21.3	*	†25.0	21.2	20.2	†12.7	29.9	16.9
							(Standard error)							
All home health aides	…	…	…	…	…	…	…	…	…	…	…	…	…	…
Health insurance coverage	(2.8)	†(0.9)	(3.6)	(9.7)	(6.6)	(3.7)	(1.2)	(5.2)	(1.3)	(1.4)	(2.9)	(6.1)	(6.0)	(4.1)
Extra pay for working holidays	(3.3)	(1.0)	(4.4)	(13.0)	(7.5)	(4.9)	(2.8)	(10.2)	(4.3)	(3.3)	(4.9)	(8.1)	(8.4)	(7.7)
Paid time off, such as vacation or personal days[4]	(3.4)	†(1.0)	(4.2)	(7.6)	(6.9)	(6.6)	(1.9)	(7.0)	(2.6)	(2.1)	(6.6)	(6.6)	(12.5)	(9.9)
Dental, vision, or drug benefits	(3.4)	(1.3)	(4.2)	(7.1)	(6.1)	(5.1)	(1.9)	(11.6)	(3.6)	(1.9)	(3.5)	(9.1)	(6.7)	(4.8)
Disability and/or life insurance	(3.0)	(1.6)	(3.7)	(6.2)	(5.8)	(4.9)	(2.3)	(8.7)	(2.9)	(2.3)	(6.2)	(9.0)	(12.2)	(8.8)
Paid holidays off	(3.1)	†(0.8)	(3.8)	†(4.9)	(5.3)	(6.0)	(2.0)	(9.3)	(2.7)	(2.0)	(5.9)	(5.8)	(12.0)	(7.9)
Paid sick leave	(3.6)	(1.1)	(4.4)	†(7.3)	(7.4)	(5.8)	(2.3)	(9.6)	(3.6)	(2.7)	(5.6)	(9.8)	(12.4)	(7.3)
Retirement or pension plan	(3.9)	(1.7)	(4.8)	†(3.4)	(7.5)	(5.7)	(2.4)	(12.9)	(3.8)	(2.9)	(7.5)	(10.0)	(12.2)	(12.2)
Bonuses	(2.9)	(1.0)	(3.7)	†(6.9)	(5.5)	(5.0)	(3.5)	(8.1)	(9.9)	(2.9)	(5.6)	(5.7)	(8.3)	(8.4)
Tuition	(3.0)	(1.7)	(3.8)	†(4.5)	†(6.3)	(5.8)	(3.7)	†(8.3)	(11.1)	(4.0)	(6.0)	(7.1)	(3.9)	(10.7)
Cell phone for work	(3.1)	†(0.6)	(3.9)	*	†(2.5)	(7.2)	(4.0)	(4.2)	(9.0)	(3.5)	(5.9)	(7.1)	(5.9)	(9.7)
Time off for good work	(1.8)	(1.2)	(2.3)	*	*	†(4.6)	(1.7)	*	†(3.7)	(4.5)	(1.2)	*	†(2.5)	†(1.9)
Paid child care assistance	(1.0)	(1.6)	(1.1)	*	*	†(2.1)	(1.6)	*	*	(2.0)	(2.6)	*	†(1.9)	†(3.9)
Other benefits	(1.9)	*	(2.5)	*	†(3.6)	(3.9)	(2.8)	*	†(9.8)	†(1.8)	(3.6)	†(3.2)	(7.6)	(4.4)

† Estimate does not meet standards of reliability or precision because the sample size is between 30 and 59, or the sample size is greater than 59 but has a relative standard error of 30% or more.

* Estimate does not meet standards of reliability or precision because the sample size is less than 30.

… Category not applicable.

[1]Provider size is based on agency type. For home health care agencies, small was fewer than 47 current patients, medium was 47–105, and large was 106 or more. For hospice care agencies, small was 28 or fewer current patients, medium was 29–72, and large was 72 or more. For providers of both home health and hospice care, small was 79 or fewer current patients (both hospice and home health care), medium was 80–224, and large was 225 or more.

[2]Includes benefits offered by the agency, as reported by the home health or hospice aide.

[3]Includes home health aides currently employed by agencies that provide home health care services, hospice care services, or both, and currently serve or recently served home health or hospice care patients. Agencies that provided only homemaker services or housekeeping services, assistance with instrumental activities of daily living, or durable medical equipment and supplies were excluded from the survey.

[4]Excludes paid sick leave, paid holidays off, or time off for good work.

NOTES: In this table, except where noted separately, unknowns were treated as no responses. Percentages are based on unrounded numbers.

SOURCE: CDC/NCHS, National Home Health Aide Survey, 2007.

Table 14. Health insurance status of currently employed home health aides, by employer and demographic characteristics: United States, 2007

Health insurance status	All home health aides[3]	Employer does not offer health insurance	Employers offers health insurance[1]	Employer offers health insurance[1]		Aide not offered or not enrolled in employer health insurance[2]			
				Aide enrolled in employer plan	Aide not enrolled in employer plan	Total	Aide enrolled in spouse's or individual plan[4]	Aide enrolled in government plan[5]	Aide not enrolled in any plan
	Number (standard error)	Number (standard error)	Percent (standard error)						
All home health aides[3]	160,700 (11,479)	24.4 (3.0)	72.7 (2.8)	37.5 (3.2)	35.2 (3.1)	59.5 (2.8)	35.2 (2.1)	10.6 (1.6)	18.5 (2.1)
Type of care provided and size[6]									
Home health only	119,200 (11,329)	30.0 (3.9)	66.0 (3.6)	28.3 (3.8)	37.8 (4.0)	67.8 (3.4)	39.5 (2.7)	12.0 (2.1)	22.1 (2.8)
Small	19,200 (5,573)	†54.4 (9.8)	43.0 (9.7)	†14.5 (7.4)	†28.4 (10.7)	82.8 (7.4)	†56.9 (6.4)	*	†24.9 (7.7)
Medium	42,400 (8,843)	35.6 (7.9)	59.3 (6.6)	†18.1 (6.0)	41.2 (7.2)	76.8 (5.4)	38.2 (4.2)	†14.0 (3.4)	30.0 (4.9)
Large	53,700 (7,947)	17.8 (3.7)	79.0 (3.7)	42.5 (5.4)	36.5 (4.7)	54.3 (4.6)	34.1 (3.5)	†10.7 (3.1)	13.8 (3.7)
Hospice only	20,000 (1,605)	5.5 (1.2)	94.3 (1.2)	66.9 (2.6)	27.4 (2.5)	32.9 (2.6)	24.6 (2.2)	4.0 (1.0)	6.4 (1.4)
Small	1,800 (481)	†15.7 (5.1)	83.1 (5.2)	45.4 (7.7)	37.7 (6.1)	53.3 (7.7)	29.2 (4.4)	*	†17.4 (7.5)
Medium	3,900 (956)	*	97.0 (1.3)	64.9 (4.6)	31.8 (5.0)	34.5 (4.7)	29.9 (5.3)	*	*
Large	12,700 (1,425)	*	95.5 (1.4)	69.0 (3.4)	26.5 (3.2)	30.9 (3.4)	23.3 (2.7)	*	†5.9 (1.7)
Home health and hospice	21,500 (3,372)	10.8 (2.9)	89.2 (2.9)	61.3 (6.6)	27.9 (4.5)	38.6 (6.6)	21.2 (3.5)	†8.9 (2.8)	9.5 (2.5)
Small	1,700 (395)	†28.5 (6.1)	71.4 (6.1)	34.3 (5.1)	37.1 (3.6)	65.5 (5.1)	33.2 (5.1)	*	†24.7 (7.1)
Medium	†6,100 †(1,947)	†12.2 (6.0)	87.7 (6.0)	61.2 (9.3)	26.5 (4.1)	38.7 (9.3)	†26.5 (9.1)	*	†6.3 (3.2)
Large	11,500 (2,604)	*	91.1 (4.1)	65.5 (11.2)	†25.6 (7.7)	†34.5 (11.2)	15.4 (4.0)	*	*
Age									
Under 25 years	8,200 (1,789)	†42.4 (11.6)	53.0 (11.4)	†13.8 (4.9)	39.2 (10.7)	81.5 (6.5)	60.1 (8.9)	*	*
25–34 years	25,600 (3,286)	28.5 (5.5)	68.9 (5.7)	30.2 (6.3)	38.8 (5.9)	67.3 (6.5)	31.8 (5.8)	14.5 (4.0)	27.7 (5.4)
35–44 years	36,100 (3,379)	24.0 (4.6)	73.0 (4.5)	40.0 (4.9)	33.0 (4.6)	57.1 (4.8)	28.5 (4.6)	†13.1 (4.0)	19.4 (3.7)
45–54 years	47,900 (4,775)	26.4 (4.7)	69.3 (4.7)	38.9 (4.9)	30.3 (3.9)	56.7 (4.6)	33.8 (4.5)	*	21.7 (3.8)
55 years and over	42,900 (5,062)	16.5 (4.2)	82.1 (4.2)	42.7 (5.3)	39.4 (5.7)	56.0 (5.2)	39.6 (5.5)	16.2 (3.8)	†9.9 (3.3)
Sex									
Female	152,700 (11,032)	23.9 (2.9)	73.3 (2.8)	37.5 (3.2)	35.8 (3.2)	59.7 (2.8)	35.5 (2.3)	10.2 (1.6)	18.2 (2.2)
Male	8,000 (1,608)	*	60.2 (10.8)	†36.7 (9.9)	†23.5 (7.7)	†56.5 (10.4)	*	*	*
Race									
White	85,700 (7,624)	20.7 (3.6)	74.9 (3.6)	40.6 (3.9)	34.4 (3.2)	55.1 (3.4)	35.0 (2.7)	8.9 (1.9)	15.6 (2.5)
Black	56,100 (6,889)	28.0 (5.3)	70.6 (5.1)	35.0 (5.0)	35.7 (5.0)	63.7 (4.7)	32.1 (3.8)	†13.1 (3.8)	22.9 (4.3)
Other[7]	18,900 (3,514)	†30.1 (8.0)	68.2 (8.1)	30.8 (7.3)	37.4 (9.9)	67.5 (7.5)	45.1 (7.8)	*	†18.7 (6.3)
Hispanic or Latino origin									
Hispanic or Latino	13,000 (2,717)	†30.6 (6.2)	66.9 (6.3)	32.5 (6.9)	34.4 (9.3)	65.0 (7.1)	†31.9 (9.1)	*	†25.6 (6.8)
Not Hispanic or Latino	144,900 (10,980)	23.9 (3.1)	73.3 (3.0)	38.2 (3.3)	35.1 (3.0)	59.0 (2.9)	36.1 (2.3)	10.1 (1.7)	17.1 (2.3)
Education									
No high school or GED certificate[8]	11,500 (2,349)	*	70.3 (10.9)	43.9 (10.5)	†26.4 (8.5)	53.4 (10.6)	†26.9 (8.0)	*	†17.0 (6.5)
GED certificate[8]	22,900 (3,258)	20.9 (5.4)	72.6 (6.2)	44.7 (6.1)	27.9 (6.0)	48.8 (6.0)	21.4 (5.1)	†10.1 (3.8)	21.6 (5.5)
High school diploma	60,600 (5,563)	23.6 (3.6)	74.4 (3.8)	34.7 (3.7)	39.7 (4.8)	63.3 (3.7)	36.7 (3.2)	11.4 (2.7)	19.0 (3.5)
1 or more years of college	63,600 (5,779)	26.0 (4.2)	71.9 (4.1)	37.5 (3.9)	34.4 (3.7)	60.4 (3.7)	41.3 (3.7)	10.3 (2.3)	15.3 (2.7)

See footnotes at end of table.

Table 14. Health insurance status of currently employed home health aides, by employer and demographic characteristics: United States, 2007—Con.

Health insurance status	All home health aides[3]	Employer does not offer health insurance	Employer offers health insurance[1]			Aide not offered or not enrolled in employer health insurance[2]			
			Employers offers health insurance[1]	Aide enrolled in employer plan	Aide not enrolled in employer plan	Total	Aide enrolled in spouse's or individual plan[4]	Aide enrolled in government plan[5]	Aide not enrolled in any plan[2]
	Number (standard error)		Percent (standard error)						
Marital status									
Married[9]	80,800 (6,329)	26.4 (3.8)	70.1 (3.7)	34.8 (3.2)	35.3 (3.1)	61.7 (2.9)	43.2 (2.7)	8.2 (2.0)	15.2 (2.8)
Widowed, divorced, or separated	51,400 (5,314)	18.0 (3.9)	79.8 (3.9)	47.7 (5.3)	32.1 (4.7)	50.1 (5.1)	25.9 (4.9)	11.9 (3.2)	17.3 (3.6)
Never married	26,300 (3,888)	30.5 (7.5)	67.7 (7.5)	28.5 (5.7)	39.2 (7.0)	69.7 (5.9)	31.3 (5.8)	†15.7 (5.1)	26.2 (5.5)
Family income									
Less than $20,000	34,500 (4,441)	27.2 (4.9)	66.1 (4.8)	18.8 (3.3)	47.3 (5.2)	74.5 (4.0)	27.2 (5.3)	22.2 (5.0)	31.4 (4.8)
$20,000–$29,999	40,800 (4,428)	22.7 (5.3)	77.0 (5.3)	48.0 (5.5)	29.0 (4.3)	51.7 (5.5)	28.7 (4.5)	†10.1 (3.1)	19.4 (4.7)
$30,000–$39,999	32,900 (3,625)	26.7 (5.3)	71.4 (5.8)	39.7 (5.4)	31.7 (5.7)	58.4 (5.2)	39.7 (5.2)	†6.5 (2.4)	†15.0 (4.3)
$40,000–$49,999	17,300 (2,743)	†27.2 (7.8)	66.4 (8.1)	36.5 (6.3)	30.0 (6.4)	57.1 (6.8)	42.3 (5.9)	*	*
$50,000 or more	26,700 (3,202)	†20.3 (5.5)	78.8 (5.5)	44.9 (5.4)	34.0 (4.7)	54.3 (5.4)	46.9 (5.3)	*	*
Unknown	8,400 (2,000)	*	76.4 (9.6)	†32.7 (10.9)	†43.7 (12.3)	†62.5 (11.4)	†29.4 (10.3)	*	*

† Estimate does not meet standards of reliability or precision because the sample size is between 30 and 59, or the sample size is greater than 59 but has a relative standard error of 30% or more.

* Estimate does not meet standards of reliability or precision because the sample size is fewer than 30.

[1] As reported by home health aide.

[2] Home health aides could report more than one other source of health insurance coverage.

[3] Includes home health aides currently employed by agencies that provide home health care services, hospice care services, or both, and currently serve or recently served home health or hospice care patients. Agencies that provided only homemaker services or housekeeping services, assistance with instrumental activities of daily living, or durable medical equipment and supplies were excluded from the survey.

[4] Includes plans obtained through spouse's or partner's employer or purchased separately.

[5] Any government program that pays for medical care, such as Medicaid or Medicare.

[6] Provider size is based on agency type. For home health care agencies, small was fewer than 47 current patients, medium was 47–105, and large was 106 or more. For hospice care agencies, small was 28 or fewer current patients, medium was 29–72, and large was 72 or more. For providers of both home health and hospice care, small was 79 or fewer current patients (both hospice and home health care), medium was 80–224, and large was 225 or more.

[7] Includes Asian, Native Hawaiian or Other Pacific Islander, American Indian or Alaska Native, and multiple races. Only a small number of records had multiple races.

[8] General Educational Development (GED) credential given to persons who passed tests deemed equivalent to high school-level academic skills.

[9] Includes aides who were living with a partner.

NOTES: Numbers may not add to totals and percent distributions may not add to 100% because of rounding, or because totals and percent distributions include a category of unknowns not reported in the table. For age, race and sex, unknown responses were imputed, and less than 5% of responses were unknown. Unknowns are included as a separate row in the table if the overall percentage is 5% or greater. The column "all home health aides" includes home health aides with unknown health insurance status. Percentages are based on unrounded numbers.

SOURCE: CDC/NCHS, National Home Health Aide Survey, 2007.

Table 15. Receipt of public benefits by currently employed home health aides: United States, 2007

Public benefits	Number	Standard error	Percent distribution	Standard error
All home health aides[1]	160,700	11,479	100.0	. . .
Ever received TANF, WIC, or food stamps[2].	83,300	6,273	51.8	2.2
Currently receiving TANF, WIC, or food stamps	15,900	3,095	9.9	1.7
Ever received TANF.	38,400	4,061	23.9	1.7
Currently receiving TANF	*	*	*	*
Ever received WIC.	64,300	5,336	40.0	2.1
Currently receiving WIC.	7,800	1,575	4.8	1.0
Ever received food stamps.	67,200	5,810	41.8	2.2
Currently receiving food stamps.	10,700	2,892	6.7	1.6
Ever received SSI[3].	10,900	2,226	6.8	1.2
Currently receiving SSI	†4,300	1,633	†2.7	1.0
Currently receiving housing assistance[4].	8,700	1,862	5.4	1.1

. . . Category not applicable.

* Estimate does not meet standards of reliability or precision because the sample size is fewer than 30.

† Estimate does not meet standards of reliability or precision because the sample size is between 30 and 59, or the sample size is greater than 59 but has a relative standard error of 30% or more.

[1]Includes home health aides currently employed by agencies that provide home health care services, hospice care services, or both, and currently serve or recently served home health or hospice care patients. Agencies that provided only homemaker services or housekeeping services, assistance with instrumental activities of daily living, or durable medical equipment and supplies were excluded from the survey.

[2]TANF is Temporary Assistance for Needy Families; WIC is Special Supplemental Nutrition Program for Women, Infants, and Children.

[3]Supplemental Security Income.

[4]Includes public housing, rental subsidy, or lower rent because of government contribution.

NOTES: For each type of benefit, less than 5% of responses were unknown. In this table, unknowns were treated as no responses. Percentages are based on unrounded numbers.

SOURCE: CDC/NCHS, National Home Health Aide Survey, 2007.

Table 16. Types of work-related injuries in the last 12 months among currently employed home health aides: United States, 2007

Injuries	Number	Standard error	Percent	Standard error
All home health aides[1]	160,700	11,480	100.0	. . .
Had at least one work-related injury[2].	18,500	2,243	11.5	. . .
Types of work-related injuries				
Total with work-related injury[3]	18,500	2,243	. . .	. . .
Back injuries, including pulled muscles	8,200	1,543	44.3	5.8
Other strains or pulled muscles	8,000	1,619	43.2	6.4
Human or animal bites	1,700	482	9.4	2.4
Scratches, open wounds, or cuts	2,800	581	15.2	2.9
Black eyes or other bruising	2,100	544	11.3	2.7
Other injuries	4,600	1,019	24.8	4.8

. . . Category not applicable.

[1]Includes home health aides currently employed by agencies that provide home health care services, hospice care services, or both, and currently serve or recently served home health or hospice care patients. Agencies that provided only homemaker services or housekeeping services, assistance with instrumental activities of daily living, or durable medical equipment and supplies were excluded from the survey.

[2]Aides were asked to report the number of times they were hurt or injured while working on the job as a home health aide and to include only work-related injuries that they reported to the agency, that required medical attention, or that caused them to miss work.

[3]Includes multiple counts for home health aides with more than one injury.

NOTES: Having at least one work-related injury was unknown for 1.4% of home health aides and treated as not having a work-related injury. Percentages are based on unrounded numbers.

SOURCE: CDC/NCHS, National Home Health Aide Survey, 2007.

Technical Notes

Findings presented in this report were based on data from the National Home Health Aide Survey (NHHAS), a supplement to the 2007 National Home and Hospice Care Survey (NHHCS). NHHCS is a continuing series of cross-sectional, nationally representative sample surveys of home health and hospice agencies in the United States. The survey includes agencies that are certified by Medicare or Medicaid, or licensed by a state.

Sample design

The sampling design for NHHAS was a stratified, two-stage probability design. The first stage consisted of the selection of a stratified sample of agencies. The primary sampling strata of agencies were defined by agency type and metropolitan statistical area. The second stage of sample selection was done using a computer algorithm to obtain systemic probability samples of eligible home health and hospice aides.

Data collection

Data for NHHAS were collected through telephone interviews with home health and hospice aides using computer-assisted telephone interviewing or CATI. The NHHAS overall response rate weighted by the inverse of the probability of selection was 41%. This rate is the product of the weighted first-stage agency response rate of 57% (i.e., weighted response rate of 59% for agency participation in NHHCS times the weighted response rate of 97% for agencies participating in NHHCS that also participated in NHHAS) and the weighted second-stage aide response rate of 72% to NHHAS. A nonresponse bias analysis was conducted for the first stage of the survey (response to NHHCS) and is discussed in the report *Redesign and Operation of the National Home and Hospice Care Survey: 2007* (17).

A detailed description of the sampling design, data collection, and response rates for NHHAS is provided in other reports (7,17) as well as online

from http://www.cdc.gov/nchs/nhhas.htm.

Estimation

Because of the complex, multistage design of NHHAS, National Center for Health Statistics staff computed a weight that took all sampling stages into account. This weight was used to inflate the sample numbers to national estimates and included inflation by reciprocals of selection probabilities and adjustment for nonresponse. Further information on the NHHAS estimation procedures is available from: http://www.cdc.gov/nchs/data/nhhcsd/_NHHCS_NHHAS_web_documentation.pdf.

Standard errors

Because the statistics presented in this report are based on a sample, they differ somewhat from statistics that would have been obtained if a complete census had been taken using the same schedules, instructions, and procedures. The standard errors (SEs) of statistics presented in this report are included in each of the tables. The SEs used in this report were approximated using SUDAAN software, which computes SEs by using a first-order Taylor approximation of the deviation of estimates from their expected values. A description of the software has been published (7). Estimates are considered reliable if they are based on 60 or more sample cases and the relative standard error (RSE) is less than 30%. Estimates based on 30–59 cases, or more than 59 cases with an RSE exceeding 30%, are displayed with a dagger (†) and cannot be assumed to be reliable. Estimates based on fewer than 30 cases, indicated with an asterisk (*), are not reported because they do not meet standards of reliability or precision. SEs can be calculated for aide estimates using any statistical software package, including SUDAAN, as long as clustering within agencies and other aspects of the complex sample design are taken into account. Software products such as SAS, STATA, and SPSS all have these capabilities.

Definition of terms

Terms relating to organizational characteristics of home health and hospice agencies

Home health care—Refers to a range of medical and therapeutic services as well as other services delivered at a patient's home or in a residential setting for promoting, maintaining, or restoring health, or maximizing the level of independence, while minimizing the effects of disability and illness, including terminal illness.

Hospice care—Focuses on relieving pain and uncomfortable symptoms of persons with terminal illness and providing emotional and spiritual support to both the terminally ill and their family members.

Geographic region—Refers to a region created by grouping conterminous states into geographic areas corresponding to groups used by the U.S. Census Bureau, as follows:

Region	States included
Northeast	Maine, New Hampshire, Vermont, Massachusetts, Rhode Island, Connecticut, New York, New Jersey, and Pennsylvania
Midwest	Michigan, Ohio, Indiana, Illinois, Wisconsin, Minnesota, Iowa, Missouri, North Dakota, South Dakota, Kansas, and Nebraska
South	Delaware, Maryland, District of Columbia, Virginia, West Virginia, North Carolina, South Carolina, Georgia, Florida, Kentucky, Texas, Tennessee, Alabama, Mississippi, Arkansas, Louisiana, and Oklahoma
West	Montana, Idaho, Wyoming, Colorado, New Mexico, Arizona, Utah, Nevada, Washington, Oregon, California, Alaska, and Hawaii

Terms related to home health aides

Home health aide, hospice aide—Refer to aides working for providers that offer home health care, hospice care, or both; are directly employed by the agency; and provide assistance in activities of daily living.

Terms relating to demography

Age—Indicates the home health aide's age at the time of interview, as reported by the home health aide.

Hispanic or Latino origin—Refers to a person of Mexican, Puerto Rican, Cuban, Central or South American, or other Spanish culture or origin, regardless of race, as reported by the home health aide.

Race—Consistent with the U.S. Office of Management and Budget's 1997 standards for the classification of federal data on race and ethnicity, the 2007 NHHAS offered home health aides the opportunity to select more than one race category. All of the following categories were read: white, African American or black, American Indian or Alaska Native, Asian, and Native Hawaiian or Other Pacific Islander.

Marital status—Indicates the marital status of the home health aide at the time of the survey, as reported by the home health aide. The categories included: married, living with a partner in a marriage-like relationship, separated, divorced, widowed, and never been married.

Education—Home health aides were asked the highest grade or year completed in school. Respondents citing between 1 and 11 years as the highest grade or year completed in school were asked whether they received their General Educational Development (GED) high school equivalency diploma. Respondents who cited 12 as the highest grade or year completed in school were asked whether they received a GED, high school diploma, or neither. College graduate was defined as completing at least 16 years of schooling.

Terms relating to work environment

Activities of daily living (ADLs)—Activities (bathing, dressing,

toileting, transferring, and eating) that reflect a patient's capacity for self-care. Aides may have provided assistance with one or more ADLs.

Terms relating to pay and benefits

Average hourly pay rate—An estimate derived from responses to the following questions: "Are you paid by the hour while working at [AGENCY]?" Aides who responded "yes" were asked: "What is your hourly rate of pay before taxes and deductions?" Those who responded "no" were asked: "How much do you earn, before taxes and other deductions at [AGENCY]? Please include tips, commissions, and regular overtime pay." A following item identified the earnings unit (i.e., per day, per week, once every 2 weeks, twice a month, per month, per year, or other). When earnings were reported, the hourly pay rate was derived using a combination of the earnings amount, the earnings unit, and the number of hours worked per week.

Total time worked as a home health aide—Aides were asked the following question to determine total length of time they were employed in that occupation: "Since you first became a home health aide, how long have you been doing this kind of work, including the time at your current job? Do not count the time between jobs or time spent on a leave of absence." Categories were 6 months or less; more than 6 months to less than 1 year; 1 to less than 2 years; 2–5 years; 6–10 years; 11–20 years; more than 20 years. Interviewers were instructed to read aloud the categories if necessary.

Pay raise—The pay raise question was asked differently depending on home health aides' length of employment at the agency. Home health aides employed at the agency less than 1 year were asked: "Since you started your job at [AGENCY] have you been given a pay increase?" Home health aides employed at the agency 1 year or more were asked: "During the past year, were you given a pay increase while working at [AGENCY]?"

Health insurance offered/not offered by employer—All home health aides were asked: "Is there health insurance

coverage available to you at [AGENCY]?" PROBE: This would include insurance that is offered after a certain number of months on the job. PROBE: Whether you use the benefit or not, is it available to you?

Enrolled in employer plan—Aides offered employer-offered health insurance were asked: "Are you currently participating in this health insurance plan?" [IF PARTIALLY PARTICIPATING, FOR EXAMPLE, DENTAL OR VISION, CODE "NO."]

Covered by spouse or individual plan—All aides, except those who gave this as a reason for not participating in their employer's health insurance plan, were asked: "(Not including any health insurance you get through [Agency], do you also/Do you) have health insurance coverage either through your spouse or partner's job or employer, or (other) health insurance that you have purchased on your own?" PROBE: Include any coverage on a parent's plan.

For this report, this category includes only aides who responded "yes" to this question and were either not covered or not enrolled in employer health insurance.

Covered by government plan—All aides, except those who gave this as a reason for not participating in their employer's health insurance plan, were asked: "Are you enrolled or do you participate in any government programs that pay for medical care such as Medicare or Medicaid [or STATE SPECIFIC MEDICAID NAME]?" PROBE: Medicaid is a public-assistance program that pays for medical care. For this report, this category includes only aides who responded "yes" to this question and were either not covered or not enrolled in employer health insurance.

Aide not covered by any plan—This category includes aides who answered "no" to all of the health insurance questions previously listed.

Agency benefits—The question on receipt of benefits offered by home health or hospice agencies was prefaced by the statement: "The next questions are about benefits that are available at [AGENCY]. This would include benefits that are offered after a certain number of months on the job, and includes benefits offered to you whether you use it or not." Home health aides were then asked to provide a "yes" or "no" response to each of the following: Does [AGENCY] offer you . . . paid sick leave? Paid holidays off? Any other paid time off, such as vacation or personal days? Extra pay for working on holidays? A retirement or pension plan? (PROBE: This would not include social security or railroad retirement benefits.) Paid child care or child care subsidies or assistance? Dental or vision or drug benefits? Disability and/or life insurance? Bonuses? Time off for good work? Tuition reimbursement or subsidy? A cell phone for work? Any other benefits?

Receipt of public benefits—The series of questions on receipt of public benefits was prefaced by the statement: "Now I would like to ask you about sources of income and support you may have received." Home health aides were then asked to provide a "yes" or "no" response to each of the following:

- Have you ever received cash welfare for families and children, which is also known as TANF or Temporary Assistance for Needy Families? TANF used to be called AFDC, or Aid to Families with Dependent Children. Again, everything you tell me is confidential. (PROBE: Please include electronically transferred benefits.)
- Have you ever received food vouchers of food items from WIC, which is the Women, Infants, and Children Program?
- Have you ever received benefits from the program called SSI or Supplemental Security Income?
- Have you ever received food stamp benefits?
- Do you currently live in public housing, receive a rent subsidy such as Section Eight, or pay a lower rent because the government pays part of the cost?

For each benefit, except public housing, aides who answered they had ever received the benefit were then asked if they were currently receiving the benefit.

All home health aides are included in the denominator for calculation of the percent distribution, whether they were eligible for the program or not. Thus, the percentages shown in the tables underestimate the percentage of the eligible population who received a benefit.

Terms relating to injuries

Injuries—The series of questions on work-related injuries was prefaced by the statement, "The next questions are about any times you may have been hurt or injured while working at your job as a home health aide. Include only work-related injuries that you reported to the agency, that required medical attention, or that caused you to miss work."

Home health aides who had worked at least 12 months for the sampled agency were asked about injuries in the last 12 months, and aides who had worked for fewer than 12 months for the sampled agency were asked about injuries since they started their job with the sampled agency.

Home health aides were asked to provide a "yes" or "no" response to each of the following: back injuries, including pulled back muscles; other strains or pulled muscles; human bites; animal bites; scratches, open wounds, or cuts; black eyes or other types of bruising; burns; and other injuries from your job.

Suggested citation

Bercovitz A, Moss A, Sengupta M, et al. An overview of home health aides: United States, 2007. National health statistics reports; no 34. Hyattsville, MD: National Center for Health Statistics. 2011.

National Center for Health Statistics

Edward J. Sondik, Ph.D., *Director*
Jennifer H. Madans, Ph.D., *Associate Director for Science*

Division of Health Care Statistics
Jane E. Sisk, Ph.D, *Director*

U.S. DEPARTMENT OF
HEALTH & HUMAN SERVICES

Centers for Disease Control and Prevention
National Center for Health Statistics
3311 Toledo Road
Hyattsville, MD 20782

OFFICIAL BUSINESS
PENALTY FOR PRIVATE USE, $300

To receive this publication regularly, contact the National Center for Health Statistics by calling 1–800–232–4636
E-mail: cdcinfo@cdc.gov
Internet: http://www.cdc.gov/nchs

DHHS Publication No. (PHS) 2011–1250
CS221530
T39233 (05/2011)

FIRST CLASS
POSTAGE & FEES PAID
CDC/NCHS
PERMIT NO. G-284

www.ingramcontent.com/pod-product-compliance
Lightning Source LLC
Chambersburg PA
CBHW080936290526
45795CB00007BA/2775